In Stroke's Shadow
My Caregiver Story

KYLE RUFFIN

Fulton Books, Inc.
Meadville, PA

Published by Fulton Books 2021

ISBN 978-1-64952-749-3 (paperback)
ISBN 978-1-64952-750-9 (digital)

Printed in the United States of America

CHAPTER 1

On March 5, 2010, five short months after I left corporate life and only two months after the official January 2 launch date of K Ruffin & Associates, LLC, I got a call.

It was a perfectly sunny day. The kind of day that signaled the emergence of my favorite time of year. Spring. The sky was a beautiful pale blue with only the hint of clouds. The air was refreshingly cool, rather than down in the bitter winter temps with wind chill factors that added insult to injury. Those days were giving way to what I knew would be the best summer ever. A wonderfully free summer for the first time in my life. I'd be able to take off whenever I wanted to. Head to the shore on a Tuesday. Drink with friends during the week at outdoor cafes in Philly. Play hooky whenever I felt like it. After all, I could control the flow of my work, and I only had to answer to me.

That morning, I was in the car on my way to a meeting. When my cellphone rang, I hesitated before hitting the answer button. The call was from my cousin Clairees in Maryland. Our conversations tended to be lengthy, and I was already running late. Then it hit me. A weekday call in the middle of the morning from Clair was unusual. Maybe I should pick up. So, I answered.

"Kyle, I have your mother on my other line. She's not making sense," Clair calmly explained.

"Really?" I answered. "What do you mean she's not making sense?"

"You may want to go check her on her. Something just doesn't seem right."

Even though Mom and I lived twelve minutes apart, we didn't frequently speak to or see each other. She was always on the move, travelling the world or just hanging with her posse. They were the

3

African American equivalent of Ladies Who Lunch. Retired and enjoying the spoils of life's labor.

By some unexplainable twist of fate, the meeting I was on my way to was very close to my mother's house. Within minutes, I pulled into the driveway of my childhood home for the thousandth time. But this time would be different. Like my 2:00 a.m. arrival fourteen years before, after my mother called me to say she couldn't wake my father, this arrival would change my life forever.

I went into the house and headed straight up the steps to Mommy's bedroom. She was sitting at the foot of her king-size bed, smiling and repeatedly saying, "Okay. Okay. Okay." No matter what I asked, she responded "Okay."

Mommy was being unusually agreeable. Yes, at forty-eight years old, I still called her Mommy. No matter how old I got or how successful I was in my career, in our relationship, I would always be the child, the youngest, the baby.

I asked if she wanted to go to the hospital. She cocked her head to the side and liltingly replied, "Okay." I had asked her this question a week before when I paid a rare weekday visit and discovered her in bed at one o'clock in the afternoon. That day, she complained of being light-headed and a bit dizzy. She refused any intervention. "All I need is rest," she said. I didn't push.

On this day, with a strangely euphoric look on her face, Mommy agreed to go to the hospital and immediately began getting dressed. I called 911 and fielded calls from Doreen, Clairees's sister, who had already been alerted to Mommy's strange behavior. Doreen, who works in a hospital in Atlanta, gave me a quick test to help determine what was happening. She told me to ask Mommy to smile. When she did, only one side of her mouth complied. That nearly confirmed our worse fears.

The paramedics and police came quickly, filling a bedroom that at any other time felt large, with all their beeping equipment and physical girth. After conducting their assessment, Mommy finished getting dressed and walked out of the house on her own power to the ambulance waiting at the curb. She had worked her way into a well-fitting pair of brown corduroy pants and a thick olive-green turtleneck. On her way out, she grabbed her short brown shearling jacket, which was proof that her stylish ways were still intact. There was no limp. She wasn't visibly favoring one side over the other. Physically she appeared fine. But that would soon change.

After I snatched up a few hospital essentials—her wallet, her cellphone, my breath—I followed the ambulance to the hospital that served as the local stroke center.

The phone tree had already come to life. Within an hour, friends and family began to crowd her curtained-off space in the emergency room. Part reunion, part support group, everyone was there for me and Mommy, the only remaining members of our immediate family.

We each came and went, spilling into the hall or in and out of the nearby door to the outside, making and taking phone calls. For the next several hours, doctors, technicians, and nurses came in and out. They conducted more tests, while Mommy asked over and over "What happened?" The results of a CAT scan confirmed she'd had a stroke, and that's what we told her each time she asked.

She continued to show very few physical symptoms. She could raise both arms and legs. She could grip the nurse's hand. She could adjust herself on the bed without help. The asymmetry of her face and her limited vocabulary were the only discernible evidence of stroke.

It was then that I began to realize that I was now entering a world I only knew from a distance through the public service announcements and partnerships I had established at the KYW Newsradio in Philadelphia. I had been the liaison between the station and all those good causes that rise up or reach down to meet people on sad, unexpected journeys like the one I was about to begin. I had worked closely with The Delaware Valley Stroke Association after the station's young news director suffered a stroke, so I knew a little, but not a lot. I never imagined that this tragedy would touch me.

In October of 2009, I bailed out of corporate chaos. One of worse economic downturns in US history had turned my dream job as the marketing director for KYW Newsradio, one of the top all-news stations in the country, into one I was driven to flee. I took a giant leap of faith and started a boutique communications business, where the only overhead required was a computer and a phone. I already had both. The decision may have seemed questionable, given daily reports of layoffs, salary cuts, and businesses disappearing overnight. But I'm not a risk-taker. I don't play now and ask questions later. I had a plan. A roadmap for taking control of my destiny.

My husband, Fred, and I are DINKS, the sometimes envied, sometime despised double income no kids couple. We had very little debt, not even a car payment. There were no insanely high college tuition bills in our future, and our retirement plans were adequately funded, considering we were still young enough to continue to contribute respectably.

I had nothing to lose. I had solid work relationships earned over twenty-five years of delivering in some of the most challenging environments. I had respect that came from working at companies or nonprofit organizations that were household names. Those two things alone would land me a job if chasing my dream didn't work out.

I traded the dense, hyperactive swirl of working in the city, where I danced around Independence Mall, weaving in between international tourists and school groups to grab lunch or the rare treat of non-newsroom coffee. No more driving to work in the morning, hearing what I wrote yesterday on the air today and knowing that more than a million people were hearing it too. But my new adventure was bittersweet. I was no longer connected to big brands that meant I'd instantly get my calls returned. But also, no more cocked eyebrows from those impressed that I, a young African American woman, could rise to the heights of marketing director for Philadelphia's iconic all-news station. No more stunned and often apologetic looks from men in dark suits when they realize that with a name like Kyle, I was not white, nor was I a man. No more dancing to someone else's beat. I would set the rhythm of my life. Finally.

Immediately after Fred and I moved into our home in 2002, we turned one of the bedrooms into an office. It made sense with four bedrooms and only two people. The cool sea mist-colored room housed one long desk that we splurged on at IKEA. Each of us occupied our designated half anchored by his and hers personal computers. The burnt orange desktop with its black frame and legs complemented the black IKEA bookcase crowded with professional books, software boxes, and pictures of our godchildren and other family. Our diplomas hung on the wall, his from Penn and mine from the University of Delaware.

Fred's end of the desk was perfectly suited for his type A sensibilities. Clear, organized, and with only a few sentimental trinkets. My end was cluttered with business cards, proposal drafts, design projects in progress, newspapers and clippings, client folders, notebooks, to-do lists, a coffee cup or water bottle, and whatever I picked up at networking events. Everything I was working on scattered around me on the desk and the floor, hoping to catch the bounce of my attention.

My messy work area was no indication of my well-mapped-out strategy. In accordance with my perfect plan, I made sure there were at least five meetings or events on my calendar each week. I started The Multi-Tasker's Marketing Minute, an audio blog that I emailed every other week to a growing list of nonprofit and small business contacts. My logo, my business cards, my website, ambitions, and attitude were all lined up for a bright future.

Within weeks, my effort was attracting business. My phone was ringing. My days were filled with self-promotion, advising clients, making new contacts—all the precursors for launching and maintaining a successful small business. The relationships I'd collected over two and a half decades of paying my dues were working to serve me rather than the objectives of my employer.

The discipline I had learned working for others was now yielding personal rewards, and the world was behaving just the way I wanted it to. The business buzzwords of the day were my real-life experience. I was molding my personal brand, leveraging relationships, learning new technologies, achieving work-life balance, being my authentic self. I was a real-life law of attraction petri dish and on the kind of high that came from believing I was in total control of everything around me.

For the first time in over a decade, I was home when Fred came in from work. And I was soaking up the love of my two associates, our new kittens, one of which spent most afternoons nestled in my lap while I pounded away at my computer keyboard. Life wasn't good. It was great!

During my career, I had learned to muster up the courage to ask questions when I didn't understand. If I only pretended to understand, my work and my reputation would suffer. If the white men in suits could amiably answer my questions, so could the white and brown men and women in white coats and scrubs. I owed it to Mommy to use the lessons I had learned in business survival training to advocate for her.

My past work with so many nonprofits prepared me to ask questions like, "What type of stroke was it?" "How long had this episode been underway?" I was searching for answers from the medical team that would assure me that this was a temporary situation that would quickly right itself. I'd heard about people who, after having a stroke, left the hospital completely normal.

I was told that hers was an ischemic stroke, which is caused by blood clots blocking arteries leading to the brain. If I had discovered her and gotten her to the hospital in less than three hours of the stroke's onset, they could have administered the drug Tissue Plasminogen Activator or tPA, which would break up the clot and render the stroke harmless.

Mommy's cell phone log was the only way I could tell if anyone had spoken with her within that window. I scrolled through the call log, searching for evidence that someone had talked to her before Clairees called her. Someone to confirm that she sounded normal. Sadly, the log revealed just the opposite. She had not talked to anyone since the evening before. This was surprising since the phone was her lifeline, her constant connection to everyone she valued in her life.

The CAT scan showed that the area affected was large. Still, my hopes remained high since she was speaking and moving both arms and legs on command.

"Maybe the long-term effects will be minimal," I wishfully shared with Fred, who had joined our group of friends and family.

Then one of the doctors warned me that it could take up to seventy-two hours for the full extent of the damage to show.

Stroke terminology began to edge out the business and media buzzwords that shaped my thinking and my language for decades. I was determined not to fall behind. I bit down and did my very best to understand what was happening to Mommy. I struggled to process the monsoon of medical jargon, asking questions of every nurse, doctor, or therapist when they nonchalantly tossed around acronyms, words, and phrases that were part of their everyday life but not part of mine. And thanks to surprisingly reliable Wi-Fi in the hospital, I started my education right there in the ER on my phone.

I learned the difference between the two types of stroke. According to the American Stroke Association (ASA), ischemic strokes account for eighty-seven percent of all strokes. Hemorrhagic strokes are another kind of stroke that occurs when weakened blood vessels rupture. The ASA pins most of the blame for those on uncontrolled high blood pressure.

TIAs or Transient Ischemic Attacks are often referred to as mini strokes. They're the results of temporary clots and are a clear warning sign that bigger trouble is likely brewing. Mommy was probably having a TIA the day I found her napping in the middle of the day. Sadly, it was a warning we both ignored.

As far as the doctors could tell, atrial fibrillation or A-fib (an irregular heartbeat) was behind Mommy's ischemic stroke. The American Heart Association attributes fifteen to twenty percent of strokes to A-fib. As countless doctors explained, a valve in her heart was not closing entirely during the pumping process, so blood pooled in front of the valve. That's where clots formed. When this particular clot broke off, it snaked through her system and turned a preventable condition into a massive life changer. For some, this is instantly fatal.

Women suffer strokes more than men, a fact I found startling. This interesting bit of info came from AHA's Go Red for Women.

Due to a family history or other risk factors, even a woman who has always thought of herself as perfectly healthy can find herself suddenly experiencing the symptoms of stroke.

Take a look at the statistics:[*]

- About 795,000 Americans each year suffer a new or recurrent stroke. That means, on average, a stroke occurs every 40 seconds.
- Stroke kills more than 137,000 people a year. That's about 1 of every 18 deaths.
- On average, someone dies of stroke every four minutes.
- About 40 percent of stroke deaths occur in males, and 60 percent in females.

I was asked over and over for Mommy's medical history. Every doctor or specialist from the ER to the ICU to which she was admitted that evening started with the same questions. Did she have a history of this or that? High blood pressure? Diabetes? Heart disease? Did she smoke or drink? I knew nothing of her current medical condition. I knew she tried smoking when I was in high school. Like the ladies in the Virginia Slims commercials, she wanted to be cool and elegant, experimenting with the vice that consumed my father and many of her friends. I'd sneak into her bathroom when she wasn't home and secretly smoke the majority of her pack of MORE Menthols, blowing the smoke out of the narrow window. I don't think she ever noticed the missing slender brown sticks. If she did, she kept it to herself. Even after she had to talk my high school principal out of suspending me for smoking in the bathroom, she still didn't seem to make the connection.

I had no one to ask when the last time was that she'd been to a doctor. I certainly couldn't recall. We didn't talk about these kinds of things. I recall a conversation back in the seventies or eighties between

---

[*] (http://www.goredforwomen.org/about-heart-disease/facts_about_heart _disease_in_women-sub-category/facts-causes-risks-prevention-stroke/)

my parents that took place behind closed doors. It had something do with a health issue, but it was one of those things parents don't share with their young children.

Over the years, if I tried to talk to her about her health, she'd find a way to shut the conversation down. My best guess was that it had been no less than twenty years since she saw a doctor of any kind. As far as I knew, she had not gone to an eye doctor, dentist, or gynecologist or gotten any kind of checkup. At sixty-eight, she hadn't even had a mammogram. Now we were starting from scratch, assessing and understanding what was percolating beneath the surface of her perfect brown skin.

Even though she didn't do medical things herself, she spent a great deal of time visiting hospitals. Her mother, who we called Joanna (pronounced like the guy inside the whale), began regular hospitals stays when at eighty-four she was diagnosed with a perforated ulcer. Joanna believed that doctors caused more illnesses than they cured, so up until then, she refused to see one. But she was strong. Even after major stomach surgery, she lived to ninety.

My father developed serious health problems after a virus attacked his heart. His diabetes slowed and possibly even stopped the healing process. He was hospitalized often before his sudden death from congestive heart failure in 1995 at the very young age of fifty-eight.

My sister, Lynnette, spent much of the eight months between her lung cancer diagnosis and death in the hospital. Mommy and I spent days at her bedside. Yet this familiarity didn't stay off Mommy's white coat syndrome. Perhaps it was because the most memorable hospital experiences didn't end well. Or maybe the roots of it went much deeper.

She knew about so many atrocities perpetrated against African Americans by the medical establishment in her lifetime that it was hard to imagine that they didn't affect her decisions not to seek care.

The irony of her medic-free life escaped no one who knew Mommy. She famously harassed, berated, harangued, and nagged everyone else about taking care of themselves. From a girlfriend's runny nose to her next-door neighbor's colon cancer, she was expert at schooling other people on diagnosis and treatment. She appeared to know what was best. Up until this fateful day, that seemed to be true. Her friends raved about how healthy she was. She was the only one among them who wasn't taking a daily regimen of prescription pills and visiting teams of specialists.

I teased her often about how much faith she put in natural remedies, most of which she saw on afternoon TV. She ate raw garlic or took garlic pills, which made her breath unbearable. She drank hibiscus tea or anything with the word "acai" on the label. She walked for exercise off and on and traded wives' tale remedies with her posse.

A tiny bit overweight, her five-foot eight-inch frame carried about 170 pounds. She was statuesque and graceful. She walked with the slow elegance of a giraffe, never exerting any more energy than necessary. We thought she was the picture of good health. Mommy never got sick enough for me to worry about her. Yes, there was the occasional cold, and her stomach rejected green lipped mussels every time she ate them, but knowing that, she just avoided them. Nothing ever rose to the level of doctor or hospital visit, so I chose to believe that she was as healthy as she looked.

Why worry about someone who traveled to yet another exotic place every year, stepping foot on six of the world's seven continents, some more than once. She'd been to Africa several times, Egypt, South America, Italy, Greece, Turkey, Australia, New Zealand, China, and more. During the previous fall, just months before the stroke, she and her travel mates ventured off to Chile and South America, going as far south as Patagonia. She was living the enviable life of a young retiree who still was able to appreciate her resources and would for some time to come.

Mommy appeared to have a charmed life in spite of suddenly losing her husband of thirty-seven years and then losing her daughter in 2002 when Lynnette was just forty-two. She was an inspiration and a source of comfort to many in the way she suffered great tragedies, yet she lived well. Some may have seen the choices she made as a lack of regard for all she had lost, but she chose her path, and all that mattered was what suited her. And it suited me to believe that she'd always be healthy, with little need of my assistance.

But suddenly and without notice, my priorities had changed. In the blink of an eye, my focus unexpectedly shifted in a way I never saw coming. The freedom of having an independent, active, and healthy mother ended like a splat on a wall. The assumptions that ruled our lives were now like a marbled liquid mass, sailing gracefully through the air, only to suddenly encounter the equal and opposite force that would render us shapeless and unrecognizable.

There was no way to know where we were headed or how this would play out. There was no way to prepare, because this was barren land for Mommy and me. Land we would now colonize.

In the space of twenty-four hours, I went from looking out primarily for myself to having to consider everything through the filter of Mommy's care. I had no children, so the role of caregiver was completely foreign to me. Like a new parent, I had to learn on the job. Only I didn't have nine months to prepare.

CHAPTER 2

Our experiences and the things we're exposed to combine to make each of us a one-of-a-kind soup. Throughout my life, I'd worked hard to identify and understand some of the ingredients that made up Mommy's soup.

From 1932 to 1972, the US Public Health Service conducted studies on young African American men. The Tuskegee Syphilis Experiment deceived men from rural Alabama into believing they were getting free health care from the US government when in fact they were only being observed and studied to see how syphilis would progress in their bodies if untreated. They even enlisted African American medical professionals to administer tests and placebo medications.

For decades, the men were told the government was looking out for them. But in truth, the government was merely monitoring and recording their slow decline.

Mommy, who was born in 1941, was coming of age during the height of the news coverage in *Jet* magazine and other publications that black readers consumed. This epic deceit was imprinted on the psyche of generations of African Americans. The suspicion this and other atrocities generated was passed down by parents who told their children that this real-life horror story was proof not to trust. Never to trust. Teaching us that conspiracy is all around. As a result, African Americans were and continue to be hard-pressed to trust the government or anyone in the medical profession. Even doctors of color are suspect, less so than white doctors, but their loyalties and motives are sometimes questioned.

I don't know how I first learned about the Tuskegee Syphilis experiments. I don't recall Mommy sharing it with me. It seemed like it was just in the air. It was common knowledge to our family.

It's almost impossible not to form an opinion about the Tuskegee Experiment. And it doesn't take much of a leap to believe that you could unknowingly become a victim of a vast, mysterious system that you barely understand. For a lot of African Americans, it's damned if you do, damned if you don't. Get sick and die, or go to the doctor so he can kill you.

Mommy was keenly aware of and often party to spreading stories of intolerance and conspiracy. She grew up during a period when lynchings still happened and when the system didn't bother to hide the pervasive belief that African Americans' lives weren't valued. We were disposable and rarely given the benefit of the doubt. All it takes is for one story to be true to make all others credible in the minds of the affected. Tuskegee was a real tipping point.

Mommy's mistrust of the medical system dominated by people who didn't look like her ran deep. The roots of this mistrust have worked their way well into the soil of African American culture. There are so many stories throughout our country's history that have left lasting scars on entire races, age groups, and genders. The Japanese internment camps in World War II. The slaughter of American Indians and the kidnapping of their children. The Salem witch trials. These emotional scars keloid. They mutate into a way of thinking, a way of seeing the system and adopting behaviors designed to protect you from another's hidden agenda.

All this was at play with Mommy and many like her. It couldn't be denied, underestimated, or ignored. Even if she never said it, it's there, shaping her thoughts, feelings, reactions, and unwillingness to comply. This was just one of many battles that lay ahead for me to fight.

CHAPTER 3

With each passing hour, hope for Mommy's full recovery dimmed. The effects of the stroke began to show. She was losing her ability to raise her arms and legs. She stopped asking questions even though she remained alert.

The impact of a stroke is directly related to which part of the brain is damaged, but the brain is tricky. Mommy's stroke was on the left side, which resulted in losing the ability to move her right side. She'd walked into the emergency room on two working legs, but within twenty-four hours, she was paralyzed on her right side—all the way from her smile to her toes. Nothing worked. She could feel sensation, but she couldn't so much as wiggle her toes.

The speech center is also on the left side. This is why she could no longer control what she said. Mommy was diagnosed with expressive aphasia. She could understand everything she heard, but she couldn't control or access the words she needed to respond. Some stroke victims also fall victim to receptive aphasia, meaning they don't understand what they're hearing or experiencing. For her, understanding but not being able to respond was a curse.

I grew up admiring my mother's way with words. She always knew the proper word for things and used them even though no one else around her did. Everyone else had lounge chairs in their West Philly living rooms. Ours was a chaise. Our shelf unit that housed keepsakes was the étagère. The china cabinet was a breakfront. She never stuttered or stammered. She spoke the language of the black bourgeoisie confidently, cleanly, and convincingly. She never insisted that we follow her example. We just did. That was how we learned to identify the things around us. Although we never talked about our shared appreciation for language, I knew it was something in which she took great pride. If marriage and family had not diverted her, she would likely have ended in a field where writing was central.

Language was also a weapon she wielded gracefully. It was how she showed off her status. It was how she kept us in line, making sure we didn't embarrass her by pronouncing things incorrectly and using low-class words like "butt," "jerk," or "fart," even though they weren't actually curse words.

But now stroke had stolen her voice, mortally wounding her sense of self.

Once Mommy was admitted, I barely left her side. I slept in a chair in her room on the intensive care unit for three nights straight. I only left to go to the bathroom, when nurses requested that I leave, once to go home to shower and change, and one evening when Fred took me to dinner to get me out of the hospital. That short dinner break felt like a week's vacation from the intensity of our situation.

During the three days in intensive care, her room would fill with visitors throughout the day. This was the onset of an out-of-the-blue crisis, so friends and family came in waves to stay with us every day, nearly nonstop through the end of visiting hours. Ralph, one of my family's closest and dearest friends, stayed with me after visiting hours ended and until he could barely keep his eyes open. Then he'd drive to her house to spend the night and return the next morning. Ralph lived an hour away in Atlantic City, so he welcomed having a bed that was only ten minutes from the hospital. I welcomed having someone by my side who I trusted like blood family and someone to feed her cat, Cody, while I focused on her. Ralph's connection to our family was so deep and went back so far that no matter how often I told him that we'd be fine and that he could go, he was not going to leave our side.

I found all the visitors comforting and a welcomed distraction. I also knew Mommy loved and expected the attention. She would have been hurt, her spirits crushed, if no one came. Mommy had always placed a lot of importance on showing up when others were in crisis. She could be counted on to pay at least one visit to friends or family in the hospital. What I knew, but they didn't, was that she kept score. She expected the same, and her friends didn't let her down. Or maybe they were just kind, concerned people who cared about her and me. Maybe that's why they were such a big part of her life to begin with. Whatever the reason, I was surprised but happy that they cared enough to keep coming and calling.

Mommy didn't sleep at all during the day. She had powerful social needs that drove her to be part of the conversations around her. It had not yet completely sunk in that she couldn't participate.

Our family and family friends have always used humor to cope with crisis, like a shield that deflects the pain of dealing with an awful situation. We passed the hours catching one another up on the people we had in common. We talked about their children and grandchildren. About trips they'd taken or were planning. Laughed as we reminisced about shared adventures. Gasped as we learned of someone's death or downfall. The noise level in Mommy's room continuously rose with laughter and voices competing to be heard, until one of the ICU staff would come in and shut the door or ask us to keep it down.

On the monitors, I could see Mommy's blood pressure rise when we got too loud. Even though the nurses might not have actually heard us, they could see the affect the noise was having on her as they watched the monitors just outside her room. We'd sheepishly concur, quieting down until our natural tendencies took hold again.

One downside to having so many of her favorite people in the room was that her blood pressure spiked from the frustration of not being able to participate in one of her most enjoyable pastimes—simply chatting, spreading gossip or correcting someone about a time or place. I could see in her eyes how badly she wanted to refute something someone said or add her experience or knowledge to a conversation. The impossibility of it all was so puzzling to her. Just one day before, speaking was like breathing. It was automatic. She just did it. But now her words were barricaded behind an invisible wall that kept them from advancing into the world. I could see how this frightened her, frustrated her, and made her angry. The ICU staff assumed our noise was disturbing to her, but I maintain that it was her inability to add to the noise that made her blood boil.

The staff never said it, but sometimes it felt like they were saying to themselves, "These noisy black people are too oblivious to understand they're hurting the patient." They tried to look at us with kind eyes as they issued unspoken reprimands, but I didn't care what they thought. I was exhausted from trying to sleep in a partially reclining hospital chair night after night. It was uncomfortable, and machines beeped all night. When they woke her up for tests and observation, they woke me up too. I was dealing with the biggest emotional crisis I had ever faced without any immediate family to share the load. What the staff thought was low on my priorities. The laughter was my medicine.

Mommy had been one of those people everyone liked to invite to parties. She was stylish, engaging, and pleasant. Her wardrobe was always a mature take on the latest fashion trends. She was a very selective shopper, who never looked like she was wearing her daughter's clothes, like the older women you see shopping in the junior's department. Her clothes were current and fit well, even though she never had them tailored.

She could instantly elevate a room with her tall dark chocolate presence and shockingly blonde tapered hair style. Her laugh was genuine and came from deep within. She bathed people in an aura that made them feel good as she spun tales of her travels and pulled from her extraordinary memory of people and places. Her effortless charm kept the invitations coming.

Throughout my life, I saw how people were drawn to her warm charisma. Something inside her, maybe an emotional need she had to fill, made Mommy a great listener. She would listen intently to people tell her x, y, and z thing. The better she got to know you, the less shy she became about expressing her opinion on the matter. But she did it in a way that never offended. In a way that preserved relationships. She lived for these encounters. Couldn't get enough.

But for immediately family, she gave herself permission to turn off the charm. With me, my sister, my father, and my grandmother, she didn't care if she hurt our feelings or stepped on our sensibilities. She rarely, if ever, apologized. She stood her ground and refused to consider alternatives.

When I left my first husband and moved back home, Mommy kept insisting that I return to the man who had threatened my life. Clinging to her strong sense of tradition, she couldn't see a way to be the safety net her own child needed. She held my marriage vows more sacred than my own well-being.

I kept her at bay when Fred and I planned our wedding. Still stinging from the memory of how she and my father took over my first wedding ten years before, I was determined to do it my way. Fred and I planned a small celebration. It was for immediate family only. The day before, I let her travel with me as I picked up my dress and a few last-minute accessories. She picked apart everything that differed from her view of a traditional wedding. At one point, she launched into a low-key tirade when she found out I wasn't going to carry a little silk purse to collect wedding cards.

"That's just what you do, Kyle. What kind of wedding are you having?" she asked as if we were planning to walk down the aisle naked.

"Mommy, there will be eighteen people there. We are staying in the hotel where the ceremony and reception are. If someone gives me a card, I can take it right back to the room. This is exactly why I didn't let you help me."

As her immediate, I was supposed take her as she was and do whatever she ordered. No charming acceptance of my silly words or inappropriate behavior. No window dressing or sugarcoating. No ice to water her down. What I always got was Paula straight up, no chaser.

I learned to accept her domineering behavior. She was my mother, and I didn't feel I had a choice. I kept her at a distance so I could do my life my way. But that distance had now closed to the point that we were overlapping. In the space of a day, I had become the voice she lost, the protector she needed, the advocate her new situation required, and more. We were undeniably connected in ways we'd never been before.

The parade of doctors continued to come through, which was another reason her blood pressure shot up. Her eyes revealed fear of what they might do to her, but even worse, fear of what I might tell them. The authoritarian was silenced, and it was up to her youngest child to dispense personal information that she viewed as none of their business.

Each doctor would go through their script, directing questions to her at first but quickly turning to me when they realized she couldn't answer. They all asked the exact same things while looking at her chart, where I assumed the answers had already been recorded. What was the point of the nurse intake interview? Was it like one of those personality tests you take during the hiring process, where they ask you the same question several times but in different ways, mysteriously finding the truth within the consistency or inconsistency of your answers?

"Does she smoke?

"No."

"Did she drink alcohol?"

"No."

"Did she have a family history of heart disease?"

"Well, we don't know anything about her father, but her grandmother and grandfather were both diabetics who went blind." I was too young to know if what actually killed them was heart-related.

I continued, "Her uncle on her mother's side died of heart failure. Her aunt on her mother's side died of heart disease. But her mother lived to ninety and was mildly diabetic. We don't know what finally killed her, a stroke, heart attack, or old age."

"Who's her cardiologist?"

"She doesn't have one. She doesn't have a doctor at all."

Mommy's squinting eyes and creases in her lips were screaming "Shut up!"

She never cared for my eagerness to tell the truth about things she'd prefer to keep private. She and Daddy always told me I was too honest, always volunteering stuff people didn't need to know.

In this case, for me, it was simple. If there was one nugget of information I could provide that would make this all go away, I owed it to both of us to share it. I am also easily swayed by the alarms raised by TV drug commercials with their long lists of side effects and possible interactions. Who wouldn't be? Tell your doctor *everything*, they advise. So I did, in the hopes that I would reveal the thing that would heal her and reset us to normal. I was secretly hoping they'd say, "Oh, it wasn't a stroke. It was a temporary reaction to the garlic pills combined with some exotic tea she bought abroad. We see this all the time. We have a quick and painless cure for that." Then shortly after, she'd raise her right arm and speak in full sentences, and I'd drop her back off at home and go about my business.

The truth behind my over honesty is that I can't bother to remember a host of lies and secrets and which versions can be told to which people. The truth is the truth. It's much easier to keep track of.

Mommy also always told me I was too scared of things. A Goody Two-shoes, too afraid of the world to make any waves. She reminded me whenever I refused to meet her and Daddy in a bad neighborhood for dinner. The night I gave in and cautiously drove to Camden to meet them and their friends for crabs, she seemed to get pleasure out of taunting and making fun of me in front of the others who were with us.

There were certain lies she was quite comfortable with that I was not. Like using the handicap sticker she got for my grandmother to park in designated spaces, even though my grandmother wasn't with her or even still alive.

"Who's going to know, Kyle?"

"I will, Mommy. What if someone who really needs this spot pulls up?"

I couldn't live with the possibility of getting caught in a lie. I had never gotten oven the time I got caught lying in fifth grade. Shortly after we moved from West Philadelphia to Mount Laurel, New Jersey, I had to write a report on the digestive system. Out of laziness and procrastination run amok, the night before it was due, I made the whole thing up.

It wasn't hard for the teacher to figure that out when I read my report out loud. "After you eat, the food goes into your stomach and gets digested, then it moves into the intestines and gets digested more. After that, you have a bowel movement."

Afterward, she called me to her desk and asked how I researched my report. I can't recall if I admitted it or even if the school called my parents. I do remember how horrible I felt. I never want to feel that way again. Life is hard enough. Telling the truth means one less thing in this world to make me feel shitty.

Like it or not, she couldn't stop me now from revealing all her shameful secrets of self-diagnosis and self-administered natural health fixes. Of being raised by a single mother and not knowing half of her own family medical history. When they asked who her doctor was, I'd respond, "Dr. Oz." She'd roll her eyes and suck her teeth. Her teeth sucking muscle memory was fully intact.

I'd go on to explain that she preferred to get her medical advice from TV doctors rather than go to an actual doctor. She would shoot me a severe look of disapproval mixed with a dose of "Don't tell him that. It makes me look bad." Her worst nightmare was coming true. I was saying things that embarrassed her. I was ignoring the "Do not make Mommy look bad or feel silly ever!" edict. I knew how visibly concerned she had always been about appearances. How she looked to the world and how her children made her look governed our upbringing. As little girls, Lynnette and I were taught to sit quietly in the presence of other adults and to never interrupt or interject. In our world, older people were in control and always knew best. No matter how old I was now, I would always be that irresponsible child flying into the house with her bangs sticking straight up and another bloody knee.

After her blood tests revealed that she had a touch of diabetes, I responded to every doctor's "Have you ever been diagnosed with diabetes?" with "Yes, her blood work indicates that she's a mild diabetic."

That made her hot! With zero words and one look, she communicated very clearly. "I do not have diabetes!"

At first, she tried to keep a tight grip on what information I shared. She has lived her entire life filtering information about herself. After all, isn't that what we all do? She had become so good at playing the role of Paula that her vulnerability had long ago been buried under layers of pretense and ideal imagery. This is one of the many forks in the road where I went left and Mommy went right.

I couldn't be bothered with the kind of superficial pretense that came naturally to her. It was too much weight to carry in a world where I needed to focus on competing for promotion, attention, and rank. The role I had been playing for as long as I could remember was that of a strong, worthy professional who could hold her own in a world ruled by white men. I couldn't risk getting caught in a lie or fabrication because the rules are different for an African American woman. I was compelled to be above reproach, trustworthy, and transparent. That was the only way I thought I could survive. It was the role I had become natural at playing.

Underneath my power suits and opinionated bravado, however, I was an insecure, fearful child who was afraid of being found out. Thankfully, somewhere during the countless hours I spent consuming self-help books on empowerment and leadership, I read that everyone in the business world is afraid they are a fraud about to be exposed.

We all pick and choose how we'll step outside ourselves. In which directions our boundaries will stretch. What face we'll put on to confront each day's challenges. And we defend those boundaries every day, often without realizing it.

My game was hard-to-deny truth and defendable reason. It was from that vantage point that I shared, maybe even overshared, the details of Mommy's past. The things she was embarrassed to admit because it showed cracks in her armor. But her situation directly affected me, and she couldn't speak. Selfishly, I needed to share every little detail in the hopes of bringing about the best possible outcome.

Mommy and I still hadn't grasped the depth and breadth of our new reality. We both believed at this juncture that she'd eventually recover fully and return to her former self and that we'd go back to living our lives just as we had.

I was in denial and quite content to be there. It was like a protective mechanism built into my brain. Like something that my mind did to keep me from becoming overwhelmed. Serving up small bites of reality at a pace that still felt painful and heart-wrenching, but not enough to take me down. Just enough to allow me to keep moving forward at a time when a big part of my world as I knew it was being stripped away.

My freedom and independence from Mommy was circling the drain, but more importantly, she was my only remaining immediate family member. There were memories and relationships that only she and I shared. Our bond was unique, lifelong, and one I understood how to navigate. I had taken our relationship for granted, believing it would always be as it was. But now a wrecking ball was being taken to the very foundation upon which our mother-daughter dynamics were built.

CHAPTER 4

Mommy's aphasia manifested itself in the form of perseveration. She would repeat words she just heard someone say over and over, believing she was telling you something very clearly. If she had to go to the bathroom and someone on the TV just said "Beef Stroganoff," she would insistently repeat "Beef Stroganoff. Beef Stroganoff. Beef Stroganoff." She sounded like a scratched record skipping over the same lyric over and over. She couldn't stop herself or change what was coming out of her mouth.

Mommy was used to giving orders and having them followed. When we didn't respond the way she thought we should, her blood pressure shot so high that the nurses insisted that we leave her room.

It was mind-boggling that she thought she was saying one thing while something else was coming out. We could tell that she could hear what she was saying, but she couldn't correct herself as hard as she tried. Watching her struggle was heartbreaking. It was also baffling and wondrous as I began to understand the extraordinary complexity of the brain.

No meant yes. Yes meant no. Every interaction was like playing a game of twenty questions. It was now the only way I could communicate with Mommy. Sometimes we were good at it. Other times we wanted to ring each other's necks. The more she pushed to say what was on her mind, the more impossible it became. Her anxiety level rose along with her escalating frustration, which only compounded the problem.

The speech therapists taught me to speak slowly and not give her multiple options when I asked her questions. It worked, but it meant paying constant attention to my own speech habits and patterns. Over the years, Mommy and I had developed a rhythm, a cadence to our communication. Until this moment, I didn't always realize that we'd asked several questions in rapid succession. Like asking "Are you cold? Do you want something to eat or need to go to the bathroom?" All in one breath. Unlearning that was part of the work I had to do.

She could no longer keep up or pull the right answer out of a string of options. Instead, I needed to ask "Are you cold?" and wait for her to process the question and then cough out an answer. Then I had to confirm that yes really meant yes or no really meant no. If the answer was no, I could then ask the next question. "Are you hungry?" Again, waiting and deciphering. Then "Do you need to go to the bathroom?" This was the rhythm of our new verbal waltz, one question at a time that only required a yes or no answer.

To alleviate some of my frustration, I had to remind myself often that Mommy was not being lazy, which is something I had often accused her of. She wasn't being dismissive or a manipulative prima donna, which were other personality traits that drove a wedge between us throughout my life. My feelings or frustration had no place because the only real truth was that the part of her brain that housed easy conversation was dead.

Within a couple of days, she began to turn inward. When visitors came, she didn't try to participate in our discussions. These were her peers, her chosen buddies, some I had never met until they walked into her room to visit. But it was now my job to entertain them while she watched TV and spoke only to me when she needed something urgent.

She began to trust me, resigned to the fact that she had no choice. At least for now. I could read her better than anyone. I was surprised by how easy it was to understand what she wanted without words. Her facial expressions spoke their own language, one I was fluent in. I read the pursed brow of her angry grimace. I recognized the wide eyes and cocked head of surprise when she heard something she hadn't before. Her eye rolls said loud and clear that the speaker didn't know what they were talking about. Sometimes I filled in the words she wanted to say with surprising accuracy.

I had also proven myself by staying by her side. By choosing her over sleeping at home in my comfy nest with my husband and our new kittens, that we all—even Mommy—adored.

Our relationship had never been tested like this before. I recalled our past conversations about similar twists of fate that befell other friends or family members. Before this day, I would have sassed back with an answer like "I am not turning my life upside down for you!" She would have rolled her eyes, and I would have rolled mine back at her. But now, without questioning or wondering what to do, I responded in the way she had been training me to my entire life. Like the Manchurian candidate, I blindly lost myself in my new role. There was no more Kyle. For a while, there was no more Mrs. Fred Weiss. There was only Paula's caretaker. I never asked myself, "What should I do next?" I knew exactly where I needed to be and when. And so it was.

Our community of friends and family had begun reading up on stroke, sharing what they learned, trying to help us understand what may lie ahead. Every minute of our ordeal was a new experience. The unfamiliar territory was a surreal place. I was present, but numb. I was on autopilot. Self-determination was out the window. The shock of it all left little room to be deliberate about anything. I surrendered to the motion of the situation, letting it carry me to the places I needed to be. I quickly became comfortable with forgetting that beyond Mommy's hospital room door, the real world was still out there bustling.

The advice I read online and heard from friends was that stroke therapy is hard and slow. I didn't know what that meant at the time. They were just words. I still hoped that Mommy would be special. That she'd muster up something in her that I had yet to witness. That she would embrace getting better quickly so she could return to her old life. But our past reality was hard to escape. My mother gets frustrated quickly and easily. After all, she was the one who taught me the regretful lesson that it's okay to give up. Just rest and everything will be fine. This time, though, there was no knight in shining armor to rescue us. My father, who had passed fourteen years before, couldn't right this wrong or make sure her basic needs for food, shelter, and a lavish lifestyle were met. He couldn't do her physical therapy or the other work required to regain her mobility and speech. And she couldn't phone it in. If she was to get better, she had to do all the work.

Her physical therapy started almost immediately while she was still in the ICU. I watched as my mother wobbled and struggled to sit with her feet on the ground when the hospital's therapists sat her up on the side of her bed.

Each therapist only spent about ten minutes with Mommy, but amazingly, there was progress. Minimal, but visible. On day two of physical therapy, she sat on the side of the bed without having to be held up. I smiled to myself as I flashed back to the time I took her to a yoga class. Mommy was never much for exercising. She was not a member of the gym rat generation like me, yet at sixty-four, she held the steadiest tree pose I'd ever seen from a beginner. She didn't wobble, shake, or look for something to hold on to. That day, sitting on the side of her ICU bed, Mommy's strong core kicked in, and she adjusted to the new equilibrium rules governed by having no control over an entire side of her body.

"Victory," I whispered.

I spent the late night alone time sending out emails to canceling my appointments and responding to inquiries about Mommy. When everyone left and only Ralph and I remained, the three of us watched movies and limited TV.

My cousin Judy set up a CaringBridge page so we could communicate with Mommy's legion of friends and family. At first, I turned my nose up and complained. "I can't imagine having time to do all these updates," I whined. She cheerfully volunteered.

Judy posted the first entry and gave me the password. I reluctantly logged in to read the comments and decided to post a little update. I'd forgotten that writing is therapy for me. It was always the best way for me to process what I was going through. So began my daily therapeutic duty of chronicling Mommy's progress for her growing list of CaringBridge followers. It was therapy for both of us. She enjoyed hearing the comments people made after they read the updates. It was more evidence that her posse hadn't forgotten her. That she mattered, and she really needed to matter.

As bad as things were, Mommy never cried. She wasn't a crier. She was too cool and cute to cry. On that night in 1995, when she woke to find that Daddy had died in his favorite chair at the foot of the bed just feet away from her, she immediately went to work. Making calls, managing the paramedics, welcoming people into their home in the middle of the night, making sure the undertaker had what he needed. Maybe she cried before I arrived, but not in front of me. She wept a little at his funeral, but overall, she approached the day like Jackie O. Mommy seemed more concerned about presenting a legacy of class and strength than showing off that it was one of the saddest days she'd ever experienced. She insisted that Lynnette and I stand with her alongside the casket during the viewing so that people could greet us before they viewed Daddy. I wasn't thrilled about it, but at thirty-five, I knew better than to rebel.

Similarly, I didn't cry, until the day I left the hospital for the first time to change the clothes I'd been wearing since she was rushed to the hospital. As I walked to my car, I suddenly welled up. Finally stepping out of the bubble that her stroke had formed around us, I was caught by surprise. I didn't cry because she was sick. I cried because it was the first time I realized that our lives—my life—would never be the same. Even if she got completely better, I'd have to watch her like a hawk. She couldn't be trusted to make her own health decisions. My life, my freedom, my dependent-free existence had been hijacked by the mother I vowed would never do that to me.

CHAPTER 5

There are many layers to why I was compelled to care for Mommy with such devotion, but since it is my tendency to be honest, I'd have to admit it is really about what I did, or didn't do, for Daddy. In spite of their tumultuous relationship, Daddy was deeply devoted to Mommy. He gave her everything she wanted. And I adored him. He was my rock from as far back as I can remember.

On those rare car rides when I was small, Mommy and I switched seats, her sitting in the back while I took her seat in front by his side. I'd crane my neck to see approaching sites along our route. Or I would just sit, looking straight out the window, appreciating the unobstructed view, not having to peer around the headrest and Daddy's head. Sometimes, I could feel his gaze on me, catching him look at me out of the corner of my eye. The warmth of his stare was like sunshine on the side of my face. I imagined he was taking me in, looking at his baby girl who was growing up too fast. Wishing for the days when I was just a tiny tyke that he could still pick up and hold like a baby doll but silently coming to terms with the fact that those days were behind us.

I can't recall Daddy ever saying "I love you" to me, Lynnette, or Mommy. He expressed his adoration very clearly, but without words. We were his unconditionally loving gifts from God. The family he dreamed of when he was a child growing up in the small West Philadelphia row home with his parents and seven brothers and sisters. We were the prize he had his eye on as a nine-year-old hustling to make something of himself. Competing for the affection of his family. Reaching with all his childhood might for the dream of being surrounded by a loving family that he tended to with great care.

Daddy was like so many parents of his generation. He worked hard to provide for us and to make sure we never had to suffer. He gave us the support and resources to create lives that were better than his. When he left home in the darkness of early morning to deliver milk or sling *Philadelphia Bulletins* onto city doorsteps, it was for us.

Daddy was a natural caregiver, born with a need to take on the problems of others. He mentored, coached, hired, befriended, and loved so many people up until the very end. He woke in the middle of the night to rescue people he loved from bad situations, that sometimes were of their own making.

I remember a mysterious call in the middle of the night. From what I could tell, my cousin William, Daddy's nephew, had gotten into trouble in New York. I think there may have even been police involved. He and Mommy drove to the city and picked him up. I woke the next morning to William sleeping on the couch in our family room.

When his dear friend Hildebrand was a child, Daddy had oil delivered to their cold house because the family had run out of oil and money.

He left an indelible mark on so many of the young men who he gave paper routes to, or hired to work in his stores. He inspired too many people to count, people I probably never met or who were in our lives when I was too young to notice. His need to make a difference took him to both the March on Washington in 1963 and the Million Man March in 1995.

He looked the other way so many times when others did him wrong. To me, he appeared to win the battle of living through historically difficult times and the repeated obstacles racism placed in his path. He was racially profiled before the term became popular. The state of North Carolina revoked his license for speeding one dark night as we drove to visit my pretend brother, Mike, in Charlotte. All because he didn't show for a court date to fight it. He often complained about getting pulled out of moving traffic for a violation he said there was no way he could have committed just miles away from our South Jersey home. As he got older, the wear began to show.

One heart-wrenching night, Daddy and I sat in his bedroom talking. That was his sanctuary, and we sat together in this sacred space until 2:00 a.m. It was the most intimate conversation I ever had with my father. Maybe it was because he was now talking to a thirty-four-year-old adult. Or maybe it was because the pains he'd suffered had finally gotten to be too much to hold in.

"All my life, I just wanted to be appreciated. By your mother, by my mother and father, by my sisters and brothers, by you and your sister." He tearfully confessed that he never felt loved enough. He gave of himself and never felt it was returned.

"I love you, Daddy. I'm sorry that I've never said it before now, but I hope you know it."

"I don't know, Kyle. I'm just tired," was his only response to me telling him how much he meant to me. I had failed the man who I cared about more than any other.

Daddy had gone from a vibrant young man to a beleaguered husk of the person he used to be. I could still remember the man I cherished when I was small. I always wanted to be around him. With him, I always felt safe and cared for.

In his prime, he was driven. He went from delivering milk to owning successful retail businesses in West Philly and South Jersey. He eagerly built a business that gave him great pride and inspired others. Daddy was athletic. He played basketball and coached Little League baseball for young brown boys at Tustin playground a half block from our home. He was so full of energy that some Sundays, he and some of his buddies rode their ten-speed bikes 150 miles from Philly to Atlantic City and back again.

But as we sat together on this night, his businesses had closed. He had to declare bankruptcy. He had become another victim of the decline of a once thriving neighborhood retail district. Now, his full-time job was in circulation for the *Philadelphia Inquirer*. He'd leave for work at 3:00 or 4:00 am to oversee his team as they delivered the papers in time for other people's morning coffee. Then he'd return home, take a nap, and go to the office to complete paperwork or redeliver papers that went missing or were damaged.

He gave the *Inquirer* eighteen years of his life, but toward the end, they also let him down. They transferred him from Voorhees and Berlin, communities that were safe and where readership was still growing as more and more people moved into the newly built McMansions to Camden. The city was spiraling downward quickly. People who could leave did, and readership, like the rest of Camden, was on the decline.

He was in his late fifties, a time when he expected to be rewarded for his decades of experience and success.

"People are stealing papers off front porches. When I go to rede-liver them, I have to get out of my car in terrible neighborhoods, walk up onto dark, dilapidated porches, and slip the paper through bars and gates to older people who live in fear every day. I can't take it."

"It's because I'm black," he said with shear hopelessness in his voice. "They don't want to work there. Neither do I." He couldn't understand why he was being forced to work in a battle zone. It was as if all he had accomplished meant nothing. His spark had left him. The promise of equality and reaping the rewards of hard work was a lie. He was no longer the man who believed that when he marched on Washington, he was part of change. He wasn't even able to change his own circumstances. Daddy was surrendering to the seductive pull of helplessness. It was easier to do that than continue the fights that raged on so many fronts.

"And your mother doesn't appreciate what I go through every day."

I was not surprised by his words. I was, however, caught off-guard that he would admit to me that it was getting to him. He was the strongest, most resilient person I knew. The person I turned to when life was getting too hard for me. That night, I had a front row seat to how the world around him was breaking him down. I wanted to take away his pain, but I had no idea how. Nothing I said soothed him. I just listened, and together, we cried.

My powerful, intelligent, hardworking father had become phys-ically frail, succumbing to unchecked diabetes and bouts of conges-tive heart failure. He was visibly thinner, and his face had lost the fullness of successful living. I could feel how special this night was. My relationship with my father had turned a corner. He was treating me like an adult, no longer the child he felt the need to protect from the realities of his life. But I had no idea how close I was to losing him.

His health continued to decline over the next few months, and so did his desire to get better. There were lots of doctor visits and a few hospital stays. But nothing seemed to change.

On November 8, we celebrated his fifty-eighth birthday in underwhelming style. I left work for an extra-long lunch to bring him a gift and a small feast of his favorite Chinese food. When I arrived, he was upstairs in his room while Mommy was downstairs, tending to some house project.

"I'm not coming downstairs," he growled.

"I brought you lunch. Don't you want to come down so the three of us can eat together in the kitchen?"

"No. I'm not talking to your mother. I told her we had a glue gun, but instead of her looking for it, she went out and bought another one."

There's no way a glue gun could generate that kind of animosity. We were in last straw territory.

"Open your present," I insisted. The shoebox was still in the bag from the store where I'd purchased them that morning. Daddy loved clothes and shoes as much as Mommy did. I had gotten him a pair of black lace-up ankle boots that I thought would lift his spirits. He opened the box, took out one shoe, and without expression, he put it back in the box without a word. I had again failed to give him what he truly needed in that moment.

"I'm leaving your mother. I just can't take it anymore. She just spends money and pays no attention to me when I tell her not to."

I just sat silently. I had no idea how to respond. They'd been married thirty-seven years, arguing day in and day out. Why was today different?

I don't remember my parents ever having a conversation. No "How was your day?" or "Let me tell you a funny story." Not even "What do you want for dinner?" She always spoke to him in a high pitch, and he always barked back. They were at odds twenty-four hours a day. Even during the happy times, they couldn't agree on anything. That was their dance, which I thought would go on forever.

Thanksgiving rolled around, and he hadn't left. I hosted the dinner at my house. Mommy came over to help because we were expecting nearly a dozen people for a snug but festive dinner at my town house. As was the tradition, Hazel, Mommy's best friend, and her husband, their grown sons, and their growing families were all joining us. Hazel wasn't well, but that wasn't unusual. She was often hospitalized or bedridden for something.

Daddy bounced around, checking on everyone and making sure Hazel was comfortable and had whatever she needed. He was like his old self, looking out for everyone else, making sure everyone was having a good time. As the evening wore down, I promised I'd bring leftovers to Daddy in the morning.

Leaving enough time to drive the fifteen minutes to their house before heading to work, I carefully gathered up turkey and stuffing, mac and cheese, greens, Mommy's signature bluefish, and sweet potato pie. I drove over and put everything in the kitchen. Mommy wasn't home, but Daddy was upstairs, lying across the bed. As I approached the room, I stilled myself and looked to make sure he was breathing. Daddy was a snorer, but his breathing was uncharacteristically quiet. Thank goodness his chest rose and lowered.

"Your leftovers are downstairs," I whispered so as not to stir him too much. He gestured that he heard me, and I left and headed to work. Later that morning, he called me at the office. Daddy never called me at the office.

"You forgot the gravy. That is what I was really looking forward to."

"I'm sorry, Daddy. I'll bring it by tonight."

Night came, and my workday ended at its usual 8:30 p.m., but I was tired. I decided to go home and not go back out. I'd bring the gravy over in the morning. I laid my head on my pillow with guilt nagging me, but I'd make up for it in the morning.

At 2:00 a.m., my phone rang. It was Mommy. "I can't wake your father up."

He had passed away quietly in his sleep. That was precisely the moment that the guilt I felt for breaking my promise to bring him gravy became a permanent mental and emotional scar. Did he die feeling I didn't love and care about him? Was my disappointing him that last thing his failing heart couldn't take?

What I now did for Mommy, I did because I never got over the feeling that I failed him. In my mind, I was the one person who loved him the most, and he gave up because I broke his heart. I ignored a simple request that would have made him so happy.

Watching over her was part penance and part making sure I didn't add to my list of painful regrets. I've blamed myself for not doing more to remind Daddy that life was worth living. To assure him that this hopeless period would pass and things would get better. And that leaving Mommy didn't have to mean leaving all of us.

I wish I could take the high road and say that I did for her because he was watching me from heaven, grading me for how well I answered the call. Looking for proof that I was using the love he poured into me to care for the precious gifts he left behind. Or I could say I was reacting to her attempts at brainwashing me to care for her. But I had found ways to deflect that by keeping just enough distance between the two of us.

I don't look inside myself and see the selfless acts of a loving daughter. My caregiving comes from a selfish place. I poured energy into caring for Mommy for my own sake. I'm driven to protect my heart from the bitter anguish that comes with not believing I did all I could to keep the people I love here. I didn't pay close enough attention to Daddy's mental state and physical ailments. I stood on the sidelines while Mommy took the lead. I didn't challenge either of them when I thought they should do differently. I didn't ask for details or give my input. I live every day wondering if Daddy would still be here if I had been more involved.

I did what I did for Mommy so I could live with myself if something went wrong. Because I couldn't save Daddy and Lynnette, I needed to feel I was doing whatever I could for Mommy. My motivation was purely about avoiding guilt, pain, and shame mingled with the fear that others might look down on me if I didn't give her my all.

CHAPTER 6

After ICU, Mommy was moved to a progressive care unit or, in medical jargon, the PCU. She now had a roommate, and the nurse-to-patient ratio was noticeably different. I missed the ICU's single-bed rooms, where each nurse was assigned to only two patients and there was plenty of room for the reclining guest chairs. In the new unit, tracking down nurses for simple things like water, tissues, or a bedpan was like trying to track someone in a crowd who keeps moving farther and farther away from you. Or like chasing something in a dream that you can never catch. In the ICU, Mommy was the star of the show. Her nurse was never more than a faint call away.

The upside was that I could now go home at night. I was still spending the entire day with Mommy, but in the PCU, hospital visiting hours were strictly enforced, which meant I had good reason to leave at a reasonable hour. In the ICU, I'd ask her each night if she wanted me to stay, and without words, her answer was clear. Her eyes begged, "Please stay. I don't want to be left alone." My heart sank for her and for myself. I wanted to sleep in my own bed, not in a pleather hospital recliner. But I couldn't leave her by herself.

After all, she didn't leave me when I stood outside my new kindergarten classroom crying for four straight days. On the fifth day, I only went inside the room because she came with me. By midmorning, I had adjusted, and she told me that she was going to visit my sister in her classroom upstairs. Much later in life, I learned she didn't visit my sister. She left the building and took a bus to Center City to shop.

This room change also marked the beginning of our crash course on constant transition. Like most businesses, in health care, the paying customer drives the decisions or the quality of customer service. Unfortunately, Mommy was not the paying customer. The insurance company was.

In the PCU, where they take patients too sick to stay on a regular hospital floor but not sick enough to be in the intensive care unit, it no longer felt like our comfort, care, and concerns were the highest priority. The hospital staff didn't come running each time a machine beeped or a patient called out. Nurses visited according to their scheduled times with medicines, phlebotomy carts, and test-taking machines. Food came and went with little interaction from the food service staff. Mommy and I were no longer people in dire need of attention. We were more like products to be monitored and managed according to an orchestrated plan to which we were not privy. The soldiers marched in, performed their duties, and retreated.

Her new room was so small that I warned guests that it might be best to come alone. In the ICU, we would keep the TV on all night. My parents had always slept with the TV on, and I knew it was a source of comfort for Mommy, like an electronic teddy bear. I knew she'd feel better if it stayed on, but I was afraid her roommate would complain. Thankfully she didn't. It seemed like something so small, until now. It was important to her, and it would have broken my heart if she couldn't get her way.

I continued to post brief progress reports on CaringBridge daily. Every day, the list of followers grew. Reading their messages to her gave us something to look forward to, something that would make the hours in the bland hospital space go by more quickly.

At this point, we only knew that Mommy's perseveration affected her ability to speak. It quickly became clear that she was not only repeating words and phrases over and over, but it also affected her ability to eat. It started when we were celebrating the first day Mommy was cleared to eat food on her own. Stroke often affects one's ability to swallow, but thank goodness, this wasn't the case.

Ralph, who had barely left our side, and Diane, my cousin-in-law, were with us when her first food tray arrived. We felt confident that she could handle the simple task of eating, so we turned our attention away from her and continued our conversation. We laughed and talked, not noticing that she was shoveling food into her mouth. With her left hand, she was uncontrollably repeating the same plate-to-mouth motion, unable to stop on her own. By the time we noticed, both sides of her cheeks were filled with food, yet she continued to shovel. We all jumped toward her, taking the fork out of her hand and screaming questions at her.

"What are you doing? Why are you stuffing your face with food? You know better than that! You're going to choke. Do you want to choke?"

She just looked at us blankly. Then came a look of wounded confusion. Our rapid-fire questions and histrionics overwhelmed her. She couldn't defend herself from our sudden assault. I took the fork and began feeding her slowly, waiting for her to swallow each mouthful before giving her another.

During therapy, she began attempting basic things for the first time since the stroke. I watched with anticipation as my right-handed mother picked up a pen and began trying to write with her left hand. My hopes were dashed when all she could write was the letter *L* over and over and over. Each day revealed more and more things stroke had stolen from Mommy and reminded me of all the simple things we take for granted.

I tried to get her to talk on the phone. I made the unscientific assumption that since she did that so often before, her reflexes would kick in, and suddenly she'd be back to chatting away. She would have brief conversations, most lasting about seventeen seconds. By her responses, I could tell that she understood what the callers were saying, but her words failed her. She'd get frustrated quickly, give up, and hand me the phone to finish off the conversation for her.

After a couple of days, we were moved to an even less intensive unit. Various doctors stopped by during their once-a-day rounds. One of the doctors nonchalantly reported that anything Mommy didn't get back in the first week, she would never get back. That was crushing news. It had already been six days, and she couldn't move anything on her right side, and she was impossible to understand.

When my sister was sick, I'd ask the doctors questions that they couldn't answer. I didn't think my questions were particularly complicated, yet these highly paid specialists, who spent day in and day out working with people with cancer, couldn't give me a straight answer about anything. At the time, I concluded that they were bad doctors in a bad hospital. But here I was again, asking questions to doctors in a regional stroke center. They couldn't answer me, or sometimes they gave me the wrong answer. The doctor who told me Mommy wouldn't recover anything after the first week was dead wrong. Later, I'd learn that the brain's healing process is ongoing. It's slow, but patients can continue to make progress for years after a stroke. I hoped that this would be the case for her.

I found it difficult to adjust to Mommy's new and complete vulnerability. One evening, her male nurse had to sponge bathe her. His name was Steve or Joe or Mike, something shortened in that manly "Hey, buddy" kind of way. He was far from your traditional nurse profile. He was a fit, good-looking middle-aged man. His hair was dark, and in March, he appeared tanned. His scrubs were crisp and fitted, not baggy or covering up street clothes like some of the other nurses. His accent reminded me a little of Rocky Balboa, but he spoke more cleanly than Sylvester Stallone's version of a born-and-raised South Philadelphian. He gave Mommy her bath, and then, while I sat in the room chatting with him, he rubbed lotion over her *entire* body.

He didn't appear struck by the inappropriateness of this. After all, it was his job, and I could tell he took pride in doing it well. He never handled her in a sexual way. Nor was the manner in which he touched her alarming, even though he covered nearly every inch of her. She didn't signal that she wanted him to stop, nor did she shoot me that "Do you see what he's doing to me?" look. But I had to look away, pretending to eye something else in the room.

Mommy had surrendered entirely to her new helplessness. That quickly, she had come to terms with others doing everything for her, even the most personal things!

It was me who was slung against the wall of our new reality. Even though I was uncomfortable, I tried not to show it. I chose to ignore my discomfort and not question the situation. If she didn't react, why should I? I had become her surrogate, mouthpiece, and interpreter. That was it. My feelings didn't matter.

I had been ignoring Mommy's personal business. But as it sank in further and further that she wasn't making the kind of progress that would send her right back home, so did the my understanding that I had to take over everything immediately. Her cat, Cody, needed to be cared for. Bills needed to be paid. Her house needed to be looked after. Her cars needed attention. She was stricken mid-stride while still in the midst of living it up. I alone had to figure out and pick up where she left off.

At her age and in what we thought was good health, she didn't see the need to share the details of her financial life with me. I had just crashed into the generational barrier parents put up to keep their children out of their business. I didn't push it because, like her, I believed this day was a long way off.

On top of everything else, I had to manage her affairs without any input from her. She couldn't tell me where to find anything or how to continue whatever she started. I had to figure out how to keep all her balls in the air, even though I didn't know how many balls there were or how close they were to falling to the ground.

I knew nothing. Absolutely nothing. What income did she have? How would I access her bank accounts? What credit cards did she have? Were there any outstanding balances? When was the last time her utility bills and homeowners insurance were paid? Where did she keep her bills? What was the status of the two houses she was renting out in Philadelphia? How does Medicare and Medigap work? When and how do I pay her real estate taxes? Does she still pay income tax since she's retired? I had to take all of this on. There would be no delegating. These are all matters she would consider private. And one of my many new jobs was to make sure they stayed that way.

The house the paramedics retrieved her from was the four-bed-room, split-level colonial we had moved into as a family of four in 1971. I knew that the house was mortgage-free and that she hadn't taken any additional mortgages out.

The cat was aging and sickly. There could be no delay in han-dling him and her expenses. I didn't have the luxury of putting it off until I was ready. Leaving things to fall apart while she was rebuilding would only result in more complications for me. Even though my goal was to get her back to her old life, it would be some time before that could happen.

When she could do little more than scribble a line on paper, I established myself as her power of attorney so I could access private information and work with people like bank employees who wouldn't talk to me without it. My friend and neighbor Marci, an attorney, popped over to the hospital on her lunch break with the POA documents. Mommy scribbled a line as the hospital concierge witnessed. That box was now checked.

After only a day or two, Mommy was to be moved to an acute rehabilitation facility. A social worker came by the room with a short list of places and asked which one I wanted Mommy to go to. I didn't feel at all prepared to answer that question. It had only been six days since Mommy's stroke, and I spent every waking hour with her. When was I supposed to school myself on rehab facilities? How could I know which was the best? What was I supposed to base my decision on? It felt too early. Like they were forcing her on to the next place before either of us was ready.

Right or wrong, I chose convenience. She would go to the facility attached to the hospital she was currently in. She didn't even have to get dressed to make the transfer. The bridge to the facility was at the end of the unit she was on. They put her in a wheelchair, covered her with blankets, and wheeled her through the doors to the place where the real work would begin.

CHAPTER 7

A friend once told me that her father became her best friend after his stroke. I discounted it at the time. Even if I thought it true for her, it would never be true for me. My mother and I had a relationship borne out of obligation. Her obligation to be a good mother in the eyes of anyone who might be watching. Her obligation to complete what she started as a teenager, the night she fell to what I presume was her boyfriend's pressure. "Just try it. You'll enjoy it."

Choice was not a factor for an unmarried woman who was with child in the late fifties in the family Mommy grew up in. Mindless obligation drove every decision. The loudest voice in Mommy's family was that of her evangelist grandmother with whom she and her mother, Joanna, lived. Nana made it known that having a baby outside of marriage was not an option. It disgraced the whole family. Mommy's condition brought such upheaval that both she and her mother, who was guilty of nothing, were kicked out of the only home Mommy had known.

The child was my sister. The night Lynnette was conceived, the door leading to whatever future Mommy saw for herself slammed shut. So much so that she never talked about what she could have been to me or my sister. Growing up, I never heard her say anything to anyone. After she got pregnant, it was as if her dreams never existed. The next door that opened was to her sealed fate of being a wife at sixteen, then a mother one month after she turned seventeen. She so strongly believed in the absoluteness of obligation that she buried her talents, desires, and needs under the presumed persona of dutiful wife, loving mother, and caregiver to family members who would eventually need her. She did not choose this new path, but she fully accepted it.

Mommy's fate was written by unforeseen forces like religion, family, and keeping up appearances. Things are simply done a certain way, and that's how it is. I suppose it makes life easier, not having to wonder what to do in the scramble of catastrophe. Never having to ask what my role shall be.

Fast-forward to 2010. The tables had turned. I was now the caregiver to my caretaker. But I was influenced by a combination of generational differences and other people in my life, like Fred. I had come to believe that our fate is our own to determine, even if we made the kind of mistakes for which previous generations punished themselves. I believed that choice, personal choice, is real and that my past didn't determine my future. Yet I was torn. Still marching according to instructions beamed into my head by my family and what I had observed. Even with my strong will, it was incredibly difficult and, in some ways, impossible to escape the gravitational pull of generations of tradition.

Who was I going to be now that Mommy's stroke had changed everything for me? Was I going to be the well-trained daughter whose role was forged in the generational fires of family caregiver expectations? Was my script already written? Was my role predetermined by African American culture and history? Would I honor what I witnessed from those who came before? Like them, did I no longer matter? Was I going to pretend that I was not suffering?

In this moment, at this early stage of our journey, I didn't rebel. I fell in line and performed like a good little actress.

She was all that mattered. I moved without thinking or feeling. I bent in the direction she needed me. No questioning. When at a crossroads, no looking for a reason to choose my needs over hers. Any comfort I experienced would somehow be stealing from her. Becoming a living, breathing martyr, sacrificing and shutting out any pain or feelings of personal loss. Cutting off anything that interfered with tending to her.

But wait. I have a husband to consider. How could I give her my complete attention through all this when I had made a binding nuptial promise to him? My heart and soul were tied to his every thought and feeling by choice. Now our relationship was up against a long personal and cultural history that would inevitably influence me. I was being pulled in opposite directions by choice and obligation, like the rope in a tug of war.

Family caregiving in the black community has deep roots. There is an assumption that children *will* take care of their aging parents. They'll never be put in to a facility as long as at least one child is alive, healthy enough, and has the means to care for their mother or father. Although this may be changing, the old ways hold many of us in a tight grip.

There were so many caregiving pivot points that shaped my behavior. I watched many play out throughout the years. Some loving examples, at least by appearances. Others, not so much. Mommy was at the center of most of them.

My Aunt Evelyn, Daddy's sister who never married or moved out of her parents' home, became my grandfather's full-time caregiver. She was a tiny woman with a Herculean will. I remember vaguely that my father and his brothers and sisters visited and lent helping hands, but she was on the frontlines. She cooked, cleaned, and managed the house and Granddaddy's needs. She was fully available to him twenty-four hours a day. If she ever complained, I never heard her. The adults in my family never shared their angst with the children. I'm sure there was plenty, but from my perspective, Aunt Evelyn was honored to care for her father in his final years.

Joanna, Mommy's mother, took care of Nana, her blind and diabetes-riddled mother. After an ugly divorce, Joanna moved back to Philadelphia from Ohio. This worked in my great-grandmother's favor because it brought her eldest daughter back home in time to care for her. Even though years before, Nana had tossed Joanna out, that no longer seemed to matter.

Uncle Jimmy, Joanna's brother, who never married or moved out of their childhood home, was one bedroom away from his dying mother. Joanna and Jimmy shared the work of caring for Nana, but as women often do, Joanna appeared to carry the heavier load.

Eventually, Mommy took in Joanna for the last few years of her life, even though their relationship was a difficult one. But Mommy put it off as long as her conscience would allow. It took a doctor explaining that Joanna was lucky to still be alive for Mommy to finally take her in.

Their journey began after Joanna had surgery for a perforated ulcer, a procedure that doctors believed the eighty-year-old wouldn't survive. She seemed headed for one of my mother's spare bedrooms, but she rallied, got better, and returned to her own home.

For a time afterward, Lynnette, my cousin Jimmy, and I looked out for Joanna. We all lived in Philadelphia at the time and were closer to Joanna than Mommy. That gave Mommy the excuse she needed to abdicate her mother's care to us.

"She makes my blood pressure shoot up," Mommy would tell Lynnette and me each time she saw or spoke with her mother. That was clearly an excuse or characteristic self-diagnosis since Mommy had never been to a doctor to be diagnosed with hypertension.

So Lynnette paid Joanna's bills. My cousin Jimmy took her on weekday errands, until dementia melted her filters and she began spouting off nasty, distorted memories of his family.

I took her food shopping, put her trash out every week, and taxied her to and from doctor's appointments. My relationship with my grandmother had many ups and downs. She was one of my favorite people when she moved back from Ohio when I was eight years old. I would tag along when she worked for Brother, making home visits to teach women how to use their new sewing machines. Some evenings, I would even forgo watching TV so I could lie across her bed and read the Bible with her. We started from the very beginning and were going to read it through to the very end.

Things turned ugly when I was an adult. While driving her home from Thanksgiving dinner at my parents, she gave me an earful about how much she hated my father. In spite of all he had done for her daughter and granddaughters, she let me know she thought he was never good enough for my mother. Her words were tinged with stinging rebuke for ruining her daughter's life at sixteen.

Decades had passed, and she had spent so many seemingly joyous times with him and us. Why is she bringing this up now? Instead of connecting her hateful words to early onset dementia, I withdrew.

I didn't visit or speak to her for a year or so after that. But after the surgery, I had to put my hurt feelings aside and be there for her.

One morning, after I had moved back to New Jersey, I got a frantic call from my mother as I drove to work. "I can't reach your grandmother. I keep calling, but she's not picking up."

Her panic quickly turned into my marching orders, so I just kept driving. I flew past my office in Camden and headed across the Ben Franklin Bridge, down the Schuylkill Expressway, straight for Joanna's West Philadelphia house. I moved as quickly as I could through rush hour traffic as frightening thoughts filled my head.

What would I find when I arrived? Had someone broken in and attacked her? Joanna lived in a pretty dodgy neighborhood, where her safety was easily in question. There was an active drug house directly across the street. Had she died in her sleep? From what? My fear and concern mixed with resentment that my mother was shirking her responsibility. Why wasn't Mommy dealing with this? It's *her* mother. Here I was, missing work while she sat comfortably tucked away miles from her daughterly duties.

Joanna's house was turn of the century. The original heavy wood front door with etched and beveled glass had a decades-old security chain that had been painted over again and again. Yet it was still doing its job, making it impossible for me to open the door enough to squeeze my hand through. I was stuck outside, unable to determine what was happening inside of her dank, old house. Even the blinds were shut tight to keep out any prying eyes, including mine.

I called her name through the narrow opening. She didn't answer. I tried the front window. It was securely locked and nailed shut, the result of a typical old person's extreme paranoia. The basement window was fastened down with a sheet of wood covering the glass on the inside. I could force my way into the gated and locked alley to try to enter through the back of the house, but I already knew each window would be just as impenetrable as the ones in the front. I decided to try anyway.

As I headed off the front porch down the cracked cement steps, I spotted a repairman arriving to start his day's work at a neighbor's house. I flagged him down and begged him to help me get into my grandmother's house. I must have looked out of place. Wearing a black pantsuit and heels, hair perfectly coifed, and my words completely free of urban accent or slang. It was 9:00 a.m. on a weekday. Who would break into a house at 9:00 a.m. on a weekday?

He surveyed me and my black sports car. It was one of very few cars parked on the block, and it sat directly in front of the house I was asking him to help me violate. Once he determined I could be trusted, he flung into action, responding to my urgent plea to cut the chain. He searched his truck for the right tool and pulled out a bolt cutter. Together we marched back up the steps and onto the porch. With one loud "goink," I was in.

I had not deemed him trustworthy enough to follow me into the house. I'd rather take my chances with what was already inside rather than invite more trouble in. After all, behind closed doors, it would be him versus my 135-pound self and Joanna's eighty-seven years of frail spunk. The odds were in his favor. I thanked him, and he went on his way.

Once inside the vestibule, I could see through the living room and dining room straight to the kitchen. Throughout, the darkness was dense and quiet. No TV or radio. I detected no movement on the squeaky hardwood floors.

The house didn't wear its years well. The walls were painted an outdated blue, somewhere between cyan and turquoise. White patches showed through where the paint peeled away from the plaster. I remember helping Joanna paint that room as a teenager after attempting to remove wallpaper. So many years later, surfaces remained uneven from our amateur attempt at that delicate work.

I started up the creaking stairway, repeatedly calling her name. I didn't want to surprise or startle her since I didn't know what weapons she might have secretly acquired. My calls continued to go unanswered.

Joanna slept in the front bedroom, having cluttered herself out of the back bedroom she'd lived in since moving back home in 1971. She was a classic hoarder. Throughout every room, upstairs and downstairs, family and culturally significant mementos were comingled with worthless tchotchkes, mail order religious trinkets, and materials she planned to use to jury-rig her next household invention. Among the mess were dozens and dozens of cores she saved from spent rolls of paper towels and toilet paper. She used the cardboard core to stuff into the sides of windows to keep the draft and imagined prying eyes out. She was convinced that people were watching her through the tiny holes cut into the slat blinds to accommodate the strings that controlled them. She had piles and piles of *Ebony, Jet,* and *Black Enterprise* magazines. Her collection was so vast that I later donated it to Ralph's museum in Atlantic City. She subscribed to *Money* magazine, which was ironic since she didn't have any money to speak of. She collected prayer cloths and beads blessed by TV and radio evangelists who prey on the fear and weakness of seniors. Her house was part war zone and part living monument to her long-passed family, stuck in a time when the future still held promise.

I slowly walked through the hallway past the layers of clothes heaped over the bannister, still calling her name and preparing mentally for the worse. As I arrived at the threshold of her bedroom, I saw her lying peacefully. I checked for the rise and fall of her chest and gratefully determined she was alive. Safe in bed in a deep sleep that was only interrupted by my touch.

I gently shook her awake, and she surprisingly didn't seem startled, even though she was prepared for anyone who showed up uninvited with a sledgehammer that she kept under her pillow. In her mind, her frail, old frame would easily lift a sledgehammer to clobber any trespassers. With the right amount of adrenaline? Maybe.

We all ignored the obvious signs that Joanna shouldn't be home alone. She didn't answer Mommy's call that day because she had unplugged the phones from the wall sockets to prevent visitors from making long-distance calls. Each trip to the supermarket yielded the exact same items, many of which were already in her fridge or pantry in abundance. On one visit, I was instantly assaulted with the smell of a burned pot of rice sitting on the stove. She had made rice every day to feed Ming, her aging corgi. Burning it was an indication that something had changed.

The mountains of clutter continued to grow at an alarming rate, yet her daughter never invited her to move into her spacious home in New Jersey. Instead, she kept up the appearance that she cared by remodeling Joanna's decaying kitchen, putting down a new floor, giving it a fresh coat of paint, and buying her a new kitchen table. Mommy left the tough stuff like regular visits up to me and, until she got sick, Lynnette.

"I'm surprised she has survived this long on her own," her doctor expressed with shock during an appointment that followed my break-in and other discoveries that concerned me. It wasn't her health that he thought would do her in. It was a careless act that would result in something fatal.

After the appointment, I called Mommy from the car and told her what the doctor said. That was the wake-up call she needed. Mommy could no longer put off what she knew a dutiful daughter must do. That very day, she asked me to pack a bag and bring Joanna to her house for a few nights. The visit turned into a nearly two-year living arrangement.

Obligation and face-saving, not love, drove my mother's decision to take her mother in. If something did happen to Joanna that could have been avoided, it was Mommy who would look bad.

The turbulence between them was nonstop once they became housemates. Mommy refused to believe her mother's memory was as bad as it was. I sometimes tried to defend my grandmother as Mommy accused her of being lazy or taunting her out of spite when Joanna asked the same question over and over. Mommy's frustration lived on the surface. It was never masked or camouflaged. Like dogs in an escalating fight, they barked, nipped, and tore away at each other. Fueled by Joanna's angry dementia and Mommy's low tolerance for behavior she couldn't explain away, my grandmother's last years in her daughter's care were painful to witness, filled with anger and bitterly nasty exchanges. But Mommy was doing her duty, and that's all that mattered.

Mommy even fought me about sending Joanna to adult day care, which would give them both a break for several hours each week. "She'll hate it," Mommy insisted. No matter how horrible life was at home, family should bear all the responsibility of taking care of family. My mother wore her martyrdom like a badge of honor. She would suffer in agony rather than admit Joanna to a nursing home. That would be taking the easy way out.

I felt sorry for Joanna and demonized my mother, until Joanna came to stay with me for two weeks. When Mommy went on one of her extended vacations to Africa or Australia, I took Joanna to visit a day care program where a good friend worked. I wasn't sure if Mommy was right or wrong. Maybe Joanna would hate it. Maybe she'd be one of those belligerent old people who had to be restrained. I had visited senior day care centers before and wasn't completely convinced when the staff said most people enjoy coming to their facilities. Even so, I still hoped it would be just what our situation needed.

While I talked with the staff, they sat Joanna with two African American women who were similar in age and dwindling mental capacity. Like Joanna, they were pulled out by their city roots and moved to the Jersey suburbs to live with their children.

Joanna immediately began to bond with the women. Each of them appreciated the chance to show off their knowledge of Philadelphia neighborhoods and church connections.

"Where in Philly did you live?"

"Oh, I know that area. My cousin lived there."

"What church did you go to?"

"So-and-so is the minster there, right?"

Joanna had discovered a way to reconnect to the life she cherished, the one that she was forced to leave behind. She was again relevant to someone, and that was still important to her. She was with people she could enjoy. People she could relate to. People who didn't snap at her when she asked "Can we go visit my cousins in Edgewater Park today?" for the thousandth time. Those cousins who once lived there were long gone, but telling her that never mattered.

By the end of her stay with Fred and me, I was at my wit's end. Even though I learned not to fight her and we laughed at some of her quirky behavior, she had gotten on my last nerve and I on hers. At the outset, she couldn't wait to leave Mommy's and come stay with me. By the end of Mommy's trip, Joanna spoke glowingly about the daughter she had not too long ago told she wished she had flushed down the toilet.

When Mommy returned, I shared our little secret. I had thrown Joanna into the pool, and she swam. Still not convinced, she took Joanna to the day care facility herself and was transformed after seeing the way Joanna fit right in and enjoyed herself for the first time in a very long time. She signed Joanna up and gave herself some much needed respite.

I took all the complicated steps to transfer Joanna's Medicaid benefits from Pennsylvania to New Jersey, and she began going to the center three days a week. On day care days, Joanna eagerly got out of bed, got dressed, and waited for the facility's bus to pick her up. The time-traveling effects of dementia placed her squarely in her past. She was back at the community center, where she and her girlfriends would meet in Philly.

She never felt comfortable at Mommy's. She'd tell me that she still wanted her own place. One day, while at the center, she fell and had to be admitted to the hospital. Each time I visited, she'd look at me, cock her head to the side, and ask, "How do you like my new place?" She believed she had been admitted to a nursing home. That appeared to comfort her and make her proud. She wanted her independence. She wanted her fate to be in her own hands and not her daughter's. Dementia gave her that, if only for a short while.

Eventually she returned back home to Mommy's, continuing her three days a week at the center and the futile bouts with her daughter. Soon after, she began asking the Lord to take her. She had reached her goal of living to ninety—longer than anyone else in her family. Shortly after her ninetieth birthday, the Lord came in the night, finally giving Joanna peace and rest, and Paula carte blanche to roam the world again.

I've heard many stories about why people make the decision to care for a family member at home. Economics is a driver. Families have done the research and found that they can't afford to put their mom or dad in a home with which they are comfortable. Some families assume that they can't afford it, never taking the time to understand the resources that are available.

Another factor is the way authority in families plays out in different cultures. Fear and/or guilt can be effective tools for parents looking to keep their children in check, no matter their age. African American parents so firmly establish the role of authoritarian in the minds of their children that a single look can communicate clearly and ensure that parents always get their way. Like Pavlov's dogs, well-trained African American children respond without understanding how or why. This dynamic is so strongly reinforced that it works way beyond the time when a parent can actually punish an adult child. Once a parent Svengalis you into believing that your job is to take care for them, that's it.

I unknowingly got a glimpse into my future when this lopsided relationship played out the day my mother popped in on me at work. At the time, I was vice president of marketing and communications for a local United Way. I had earned the reputation of being a workaholic. I was consistently one of the first in every day and last out every night. During our weekly leadership meetings with the other VPs and the president, I felt and behaved with the confidence of someone in my position. Equipped with my well-thought-out proposals, outlines, and plans, I steered the organization toward projects and people I thought would help us accomplish our goals. I owned my successes and my failures, presenting lessons learned so as to not repeat mistakes.

One day, during one of our meetings, the president's office door opened, and in walked the grande dame, my mother. My adult-sized confidence left the room as soon as Mommy entered. There wasn't room in there for it and her. In a flash, I was eight years old again. In front of my peers and boss, I began to react as if I'd been caught doing something wrong.

"What time are you getting off?" she asked matter-of-factly.

"I don't know, Mommy. Why?"

"It's almost five. Can you leave now? We want to go to dinner."

"Okay, Mommy. Give me a minute. I'll get my things." I walked out mid-meeting, shut down my computer, and turned off my office lights, and like a baby duckling, I waddled out of the building behind my mother as my coworkers watched with surprise. I was under the influence of my Svengali. I felt myself slip away, and I couldn't stop it. I don't even eat dinner that early.

In our conversations about her eventual elder care, Mommy made it clear from the very start that she intended to pass quietly in her sleep in the larger of my two guest bedrooms. It didn't matter that when and where she departed. Her natural life was not up to her. She had a plan, and like her children, the cosmic universe would just comply. She also couldn't control whether she'd get to age and pass on in my home. That decision was squarely in the hands of my husband and me. This is where my two worlds collided.

My husband's parents lived for their children, which was in stark contrast from my upbringing. My parents (more my mother) expected to be repaid for raising me. My Jewish in-laws, on the other hand, were of the "I don't want to be a burden" variety. They dutifully moved themselves into a nursing home when it became obvious that they could no longer safely live in their own house. The situation wasn't without its emotional bumps and bruises, but moving in with one of their four children was never an option.

My sisters-in-law, who were responsible for their parents' care outside the home, always remarked how much I did for my mother after her stroke. I found their comments curious. I didn't know any other way. To give myself over to her needs completely was the expectation I grew up with. Anything less would be selfish. Good people are not selfish, and I considered myself a good person.

I make the distinction a cultural one because of my Jewish therapist's stunned reaction when I said, "I'm not in control of my situation with my mother. I have to do what she wants. What I want doesn't matter." Her eyes popped wide with disbelief as I explained that in African American families, parents have complete authority until the day they die and maybe even after they're gone. This was a concept I never had to explain to any of my African American friends.

My therapist stopped mid-session and asked me to educate her. Apparently, many Jewish children are encouraged to question authority. That blew me away, even though I'd been married to a Jewish man for over a decade. I just thought he and his family were unusual in how they took pride in challenging and even bringing down authority. Challenging everything and everyone was a brain sport. Every year at the Thanksgiving dinner table, our nephews and niece confidently argued their side, never compelled to acquiesce, or back down to the elders at the table.

I began seeing the therapist because of my mother, but now my husband's position that I always gave my mother more than I was required came into focus. The experiences that shaped our lives were very different. I was beginning to imagine a world where I had a choice. Where I did matter. But years and years of ingrained submission would take work and time to undo.

I like trying to dissect relationships and apply cause and effect, whether I'm right or wrong. That's my brain sport. In trying to understand the complexities of how we approach caregiving for an ailing parent, so many things dictate the extent to which we'll surrender control of our time, resources, and priorities. Some family relationships are close, and parents and children are friends. Some families go through the motions because they've never been given permission or given themselves permission to choose how they'll navigate this journey.

For me, obligation and honoring commitments was the centrifugal force that kept our family together.

CHAPTER 8

Pity was also a powerful force that influenced my decisions about caregiving.

My pity party for Mommy started when Daddy passed away. Until he died, she always had a safety net no matter what. He rescued her from herself often. He gave in to her demands frequently. He even made sure she'd be well taken care of if he died. Her arrested development at seventeen meant she never had to completely rely on herself to meet her own basic needs. Even now, she was the teenage girl who expected to be cared for by those around her.

My sister, Lynnette, passed away at forty-three. "No parent should ever lose a child" became something Mommy and I heard repeatedly. We watched my sister deteriorate quickly after being diagnosed with lung cancer. It was a short eight months between her diagnosis and death. I, the daughter Mommy often referred to as the cold one, understood how much this had to devastate and maybe even weakened her.

These two things made it easy for me to surrender to her belief that my place was to take care of her. Before the stroke, I had already begun in some ways, even as I tried to keep my distance. If she carelessly let a bill go unpaid, she'd call me and ask me to pay it online without understanding what that meant. Instead of writing a check before it was late and putting it into the mailbox that was right outside her front door, she'd call me to fix things. Rather than buy a new car because the 1996 Isuzu Rodeo with 170,000 miles on it broke down and stranded her on I-95 in Philadelphia, she'd just borrow my car, expecting me to make other arrangements to get to work. Rather than letting me pay someone to clean the gutters on her two-story house, she cancelled the appointment and told me, "You can spend your money on me some other way. Now come over and help me clean my gutters." I refused that demand, and for the record, nobody in their sixties should climb two stories up a ladder to clean gutters.

With Daddy and Lynnette gone, responding to her demands and whims was now fully on my shoulders. There was no one to share the load.

According to her scorebook, it was my duty to repay her for all she had done for me. All the meals she ever prepared. All the times she took me to school when I missed the bus or picked me up from a late track meet. All the clothes she bought me. I would have to pay for the labor pains and 2:00 a.m. feedings. For diaper changes and consistently having a roof over my head. For letting me drive her car and paying for college. She had kept a running tab, and she expected to collect.

But I matter too. I didn't want to get lost in the process of care-giving. Every life is precious, even mine. People say that about babies and children, but when we become adults, we stop honoring our preciousness. We become workhorses, pack mules who have no value unless we're suffering or serving others.

Now, thanks to my therapist and sisters-in-law, I understood that there was another way. I had a choice. I began to wonder, "Is suffering more important than being happy?" I needed to make sense of conflicting philosophies that were doing battle within me. My experiences were so blended that I couldn't rely on blindly following one culture's tradition. My family of origin was African American, and inside me were the collective experiences and history of genera-tions that came before. Yet I'd spent so much of my life outside the African American community looking in. I grew up in a predomi-nantly white New Jersey town. I graduated from a predominantly white university. I worked in predominantly white organizations and companies. I had more white friends than black. I married white men. My white friends' parents didn't want to be burdens.

Then there was my religious indoctrination. The argument for martyrdom came from my family roots. We were Baptists, baptized in the sea of suffering with no shoreline in sight. In Bible school, I heard over and over the stories of martyrs. Jesus selflessly suffered for our sins. The apostles traded their worldly possessions for a life of poverty and, oftentimes, brutality in the name of our Lord. Saints Peter and Paul were beaten, starved, thrown in with lions, walked through fire, sailed turbulent seas and more to share God's Word with people of foreign lands. Even Moses, when he asked "Why me?" God wouldn't take no for an answer.

I've studied the Bible. I've read it from cover to cover several times because I wanted to read God's Word free of anyone else's interpretation. It took five readings to feel like I understood what it really meant, at least what it meant to me. I also know the extraordinary power of words. I've spent my life using words to shape people's thoughts, opinions, and actions.

I see the Bible and similar doctrines as the absolute greatest instruments of manipulation. Religion helps us ascribe meaning to our lives. The Bible tells us what to value and when to rise up against our foes. Those who claim intimate knowledge of the Word wield its power like a sword. Striking down opposing thoughts with carefully selected passages taken out of context and magnified by the willing assistance of widespread ignorance of the full Bible text. Even fewer of us know what's written in the books that never made it into the Bible.

I believe my family's blind connection to the Bible's self-sacrificing messages date back to the need for our slave ancestors to find comfort and value in their cruel, senseless world. A world where their humanness was ignored, where they were punished for showing any sign of noncompliance. To stay safe, alive, and to feel value, they were brainwashed by slave owners into believing their captivity was sanctioned by God. How else do you stay sane under the tyrannical rule of a self-righteous master? How do you go on if you believe your life is worth nothing?

The more we suffered, the better people we were in God's eyes. Generation after generation of African Americans internalized New Testament's depictions of what it meant to be a good person. Suffering earns us a cozy little spot in heaven after enduring the heinous struggle of life on earth. That's the logic slave owners used to keep our ancestors in line. The birth of my culture lies within the bloody and painfully reinforced relationship between slave and master. These lessons became the enduring framework for how African American mothers control and show love for their children to this day. Long after slavery has ended, few things rank higher in a God-fearing African American home than New Testament Bible verses that urge children to suffer and submit.

> "Children obey your parents in the Lord, for this is right. 'Honor your father and mother'—which is the first commandment with a promise—that it may go well with you and that you may enjoy long life on the earth.'" (Ephesians 6:1–3 NIV)
>
> "Give proper recognition to those widows who are really in need. But if a widow has children or grandchildren, these should learn first of all to put their religion into practice by caring for their own family and so repaying their parents and grandparents, for this is pleasing to God." (1 Timothy 5:3–4 NIV)

The Old Testament isn't short on messages that paint a frightening picture for anyone who disobeys their parents.

> "The eye that mocks a father, that scorns obedience to a mother, will be pecked out by the ravens of the valley, will be eaten by the vultures." (Proverbs 30:17 NIV)

Ouch!

The authors of the Bible understood well that fear and guilt are effective tools for control. Faith dictates that we push aside rational thinking and replace it with emotional reactivity driven by that fear.

Fear and guilt also lead to resentment, anger, and depression. It's like that boss you hate because he pushes you around and treats you as though you and your opinion don't matter. You know he's wrong, but you're afraid if you speak up for yourself, you'll get fired from the job you despise. You hate your job and yourself for putting up with it. You feel helpless, hopeless, and out of control.

My relationship with my mother wasn't much different. She wouldn't fire me, but she sure would make my life miserable if she didn't get her way.

With her, I spent so much time in the emotional reaction zone of fear and guilt that it was impossible to step back and see the true nature of our relationship. Interactions were defensive battles, each of us protecting what we perceived as our right to be valued and taken care of. Our right to control our own lives, even if it meant usurping control of someone else's.

To defend my space, I lashed out at my mother often. I said things that were hurtful. I snapped no to so many requests, even though I eventually granted them. Like the many times she asked me to take her to drop off her aging SUV at the repair shop because she refused to buy a new one. I'd start with no, which gave way to me lecturing her about why it was time to get rid of it. Then I'd check my calendar to see if I could manage her request. If I could, I did, but not without an attitude and a parting shot about how selfish she was for allowing her irresponsibility to bleed into my life.

I punished her with attitude the way she punished me, and her mother punished her and so on. But the stroke meant that now I was the parent, and unfortunately for her, my reflex was to give what I had gotten and what I had witnessed. I also knew enough to realize that continuing like this wouldn't be good for either of us.

Therapy helped me peel back my family's onion. The first time I sought therapy was after Daddy died. Part of the reason I needed a professional therapist was to resolve the anger I had toward her for not taking better care of him. I crossed a line when I accused her of killing him, which struck her harder than anything I'd ever said to her.

When Lynnette died, I needed help coming to terms with being the only person left to care for my grandmother and mother. During those sessions, my therapist walked me through the process of understanding who my mother really was. How her life had shaped her, our relationship, and her relationships with her mother and evangelical grandmother.

I spent hours deconstructing Mommy to figure out what was really at play in our relationship. I learned how to consciously call upon the knowledge that when we were together, it was never just me and her in the room. So was Nana, my domineering great-grandmother. Hellfire and brimstone were her brand. She was strict and quick to punish. When Lynnette and I were small, she babysat us at the dark, silent, and modestly furnished house Mommy grew up in. On occasion, my cousins Clairees and Doreen would join us there. Nana was old, blind from diabetes, and feeble, yet she still commanded our obedience. No running. No going shoeless on the hardwood floors. No loud noises. And on Sundays, definitely no listening or dancing to the devil's music. I don't recall the big black and white TV in the living room ever being on or even the sound of a radio.

My memories of Nana are of a cruel, harsh, and omnipotent presence that everyone, including the adults, feared. When we were all in bed in the back bedroom, whispering under the covers, she'd yell at us to be quiet from the front bedroom of the long, narrow row house.

"I hear you back there. Now go to sleep and stop your chattering."

My bitter grandmother was also in the room with Mommy and me. Joanna's first husband left her while she was still pregnant with my mother. From what I recall from whispers in 1970, when Joanna came to live with us after moving back from Ohio, her second husband, Pete, burned their house down in an attempt to kill her. My grandmother's life had its ups and downs. It was the downs that hovered over her relationship with her only child.

When dementia took over, Joanna was no longer able to hide her resentment toward my mother. She blamed my mother for the fact that her life turned out so miserably. My grandmother's dementia warped her memories, often tilting them toward the negative with her starring as the victim. I never knew whether the intense anger in her waning years was real or fabricated by her dying brain. But even before dementia set in, Joanna's feelings about my father were ever present in their relationship. Mommy had to live with that knowledge while staying true to the commitment she made the day she said "I do." To her, that promise was rock solid, never to be undone by anything short of "till death do us part."

Mommy quietly suffered wounds from so many others who had scarred her heart. Some I knew. Others I didn't, like the father she erased from existence.

Through therapy, I could finally process some of the things that were hiding in the shadows, that things were never talked about or explained. I could now put her into context. I learned how to look at her with sympathy rather than with resentment for someone who was a burden.

Therapy opened my eyes to the sacrifices she believed she made and the burdens she carried. Mommy did what she felt she must to honor the commitment she made when she unexpectedly became a wife and mother. She took her punishment and paid for her indiscretion without outwardly questioning whether or not she deserved it.

It was this legacy that she passed on to me, the overdeveloped sense of obligation and commitment, from which she was now benefiting. The cycle was complete. The spoken and unspoken were guiding me, and I placed my faith in the hope that my suffering would be rewarded.

My sessions and the realizations that came from them took some of the sting out of our relationship. They helped me put words to feelings and apply meaning to seemingly mysterious actions. Therapy gave me tools to calm myself and rules for walking away.

But it didn't answer one very important question I lived with. Even though we looked like the perfect family on the surface, Mommy's past seemed to scar my sister and me so much that neither of us had or wanted to have children. I never understood why I didn't have that internal yearning for motherhood. I thought maybe I was missing the mommy gene. I felt flawed but resolute in my decision to go through life childless. I never fantasized about being a mother. My sister and I never talked about being aunts or asked each other when we were going to take that leap. No matter how many people asked when or why I didn't have children, I was very comfortable answering, "I don't want them. They're a lot of responsibility, and I'm not up for it." No number of gasps or mouths gaping open would change my mind. It remained a mystery, until Mommy revealed something much later during our nearly three-year journey.

CHAPTER 9

While watching a man swim in the ocean parallel to the shore-line, I saw the perfect metaphor for caregiving. The ocean is so large compared to a tiny human. The waves, before they broke, were giant swells that looked as if they were going to overtake the swimmer, drag him beneath the surface, and drown him. But instead, with each swell, the swimmer rose and fell, drifting on the ever-changing surface, never losing the rhythm of his arm stride. He stayed parallel to the shoreline as he lifted and lowered, lifted and lowered, lifted and lowered.

Caring for Mommy was like that. As each transition occurred or a new crisis emerged, it felt as if the giant wave of angst was going to overtake me. I expected to drown in a sea of impossible situa-tions, pulled under by the weight of fear and complexity. But when each crisis came, the wave lifted me up to the place where solutions dwelled and lowered me back down to a calm place, into a short-lived routine, which was often, and without advance notice, dis-rupted again and again.

Acute rehab was the first of Mommy's four-phase recovery pro-cess. The rooms of the rehab facility were painted in light pastels and cream colors. Each accommodated two patients with beds that had long institutional fluorescent lights hanging above the headboard. Each patient had a unit that combined drawers, a mirror and counter, and a small closet. The space was clean and tidy but extremely tight for something a person was expected to live in for the next month.

I immediately began decorating her room with all her cards, stuffed animals, and flowers, like a mother decorating her daughter's new dorm room. I tried to fill it with things that reminded her of her life just two short weeks before. Books I found at the side of her bed, clothes from her closet, pictures of her traveling.

Her room overlooked the rooftop jungle gym for kids in the medical day care and rehab that was also in the building. It was March. Still too cold for children to use it, but visitors with children took advantage of the distraction, climbing, hopscotching, and whirling around on the small carousel.

There was a large reclining chair that patients could sit in when they weren't in bed. The room barely accommodated one guest chair, but we tried to squeeze it in because she had so many visitors, many of whom were her age or older. It would be inconsiderate to make them stand. I often tried to make myself comfortable on the bed, sitting up so it didn't appear that I was taking advantage. Mommy spent most of her time in the room in a wheelchair along the window side of the bed, where there was the most space.

The cumbersome recliner was available for me or other guests, but it had to be moved around and out of the way whenever a doctor, nurse, technician, or nurse's aide came in to complete one of many tasks. Because it was revealed that she had high blood pressure, borderline diabetes, A-fib, and issues with blood clotting, their visits were frequent. A constant parade of techs and nurses came in to draw blood, take her blood pressure, and test her sugar. Once they removed the catheter, the nurse's aide had to maneuver through the room to take her to the bathroom, which was extremely large with a doorway wide enough to accommodate the widest of wheelchairs.

Moving to acute rehab meant the real hard work was about to begin. In the hospital, a therapist only spent about ten to fifteen minutes with her. In acute rehab, she'd have to endure up to four hours of therapy six days a week.

Mommy wasn't the kind of person who regularly worked out. She'd taken up walking with her girlfriends, but that was more social than exercise. Thanks to her genetics, half of which was completely unknown, she was in good shape for a sixty-eight-year-old. She fancied herself a dainty lady who barely bent her knees and pointed her toes when on the rare occasion she needed to run. She ran like a movie star with cameras rolling, driven by a need to appear glamorous.

Mommy didn't understand the mechanics of repetition and muscle memory. She wasn't familiar with biophysics or how the brain learns. It wasn't easy educating her about these things either because, in her mind, she knew everything. Mommy was like a teenager who refuses to believe their parents' dictates are based on proven knowledge instead of the desire to deny their child what they want.

When the speech therapist asked her to say something simple, like saying "My name is Paula" out loud, she'd roll her eyes and give a look that said "This is ridiculous." I know how to say my name. But in truth, she was no longer capable of saying a mindlessly easy phrase that she had repeated over and over once she mastered it as a child. Eventually, she'd give in, try, and was surprised each time by how difficult it was to say whatever she wanted on demand.

When occupational and physical therapists explained why they had her do certain things, it made total sense to me. I was a star athlete in high school and a lifelong gym rat. I knew the benefits of repetition and how to build strength because I had lived it. In late-night, marijuana-fueled debates in college, I had learned from one of my closest friends, Flavia, the PhD candidate in psychology, about how the brain develops grooves that store the memories of repeated motion and experience. That's how we do things without having to think about them.

The practices I read about in my Psychology 101 textbooks at University of Delaware and altered state theoretical debates now meant something. In college, I wondered, "Will I ever need this information?" I imagined I'd need to tap into what I'd learned sometime during my career, not in my personal life. But here I was, trying to explain to my sixty-year-old mother how the brain, her brain, worked. She wasn't buying it.

Mommy never went to college. She dropped out of high school in her senior year to have my sister, yet she still believed herself to be wise, worldly, and well-educated. She knew everything she needed to know about successfully navigating life. After all, she watched *Dr. Oz* and *The Doctors* every day. Beside her bed, she kept books about herbal remedies and preventative health that would tell her what she needed to know, but I couldn't tell if she ever bothered to read them.

To her, that was enough for her to hold her own against anyone with a medical degree.

I tried to explain why it was important that she do things she considered childish. That she needed to relearn what she took for granted two short weeks ago. Why walking, writing, and talking—things she previously did without effort—would require the intensity of an athlete in training.

"Mommy," I said, "this is going to be the hardest thing you've ever done in your entire life." I tried to give her mental tools she could use to work past the point where she'd normally give up. "All I ask is when you get to the point where you don't think you can do it anymore, please try one more time."

Every day, I had to convince her to fight harder than I'd seen her fight for anything. And when there were setbacks, I had to remind myself regularly to pull back on my reflex to respond with criticism or anger. I took great pains to encourage her and support her recovery with my words and body language. This was a very different dynamic for our relationship, but one the therapists convinced me was important if I wanted her to get better. Since I was still operating on the premise that she'd make a one hundred percent recovery, I followed their advice.

It seemed to work, but there's a thin line between motivation and nagging. For me to stay on the good side of this line required a keen awareness of self and of others. I needed to pull out another lesson I learned in college about fluctuating relationship dynamics and the end goal. As an organizational communications major, I fell in love with the art of interpersonal communication, and now I had to put what I learned in the classroom to work in a one-on-one relationship with my own mother.

Three things lie at the center of communication: the sender, the receiver, and filters. We send and receive information through the filters constructed by our unique life experiences. We *all* do this all the time. Not just verbally but nonverbally too. Our bodies give away our true feelings, even when our words say something different. Something as seemingly unrelated as the condition of the clothes we are wearing or the neatness of our hair has an impact on the credibility of message.

And with each person we speak with, the equation changes. Something as simple as who is in the room when we speak can determine if what we intend to communicate actually gets through.

As for Mommy, the filter she communicated through was always "I'm your mother. I know more than you!" To open her mind to whatever I had to say, I first had to show respect for her real or assumed knowledge. It was hard work to not belittle the wives' tales and hair-brained remedies I knew she considered legitimate. It was also hard to convince her that rest wasn't the answer. Only hard work, the kind she was completely unaccustomed to, would get her back to her old life.

I also had to learn to praise her, which was something I was not used to. Praise doesn't come naturally to me. I didn't grow up getting it, so I didn't know how to give it.

In my family, praise usually came from a third party, from a friend or family member who'd say, "Your mother is very proud of you. She talks about you all the time." I couldn't help but see this as bragging rather than praising. It was her taking credit for my success. If not, why didn't she ever tell me that she was proud of me like she told her friends?

She loved receiving praise herself, going as far ordering me, Daddy, and Lynnette to say something nice about her. But usually, she had to snatch praise as it slid out of the side of my mouth when after making a string of bad decisions, she finally did right by me. Like when I finally told her she'd done good the night she showed up in my driveway in her new Mercedes.

I was much more familiar with sarcastic criticism. Our family had mastered it and were quite comfortable delivering it. But I can say, without an inkling of doubt, that you never get totally comfortable being on the receiving end of your mother's sarcastic statements about your clothes, hair, decisions, or choice of friends. But that was our way, and I knew how to navigate it.

If she was to get better, the therapists said, celebrating her accomplishments, no matter how small, was key. I swallowed my inclination to tell her that I knew she could do better. That she couldn't afford to be her usual lazy self. Or that if she was to get her old life back, she couldn't be the person who only does what she feels like doing. Instead, whenever I got reports of progress, I smiled and congratulated her as genuinely as I could.

The medical staff tended to speak to her in ways she thought was demeaning and patronizing. They spoke slowly and louder than normal. Her responses were typical of someone being talked down to. She'd respond with an incredulous look, her expression stating clearly, "Who do you think you're talking to?" Or "Of course I can write my name. Why should I have to show you that I can?" When she was physically tired, she gave her "not again" look followed by a very audible "harrumph."

"No" became her favorite word. She was slow to comprehend, but quick to refuse. If I asked a question to which the answer was ultimately yes, she'd automatically start with no before taking the time to understand what I had asked. Armed with that knowledge, my challenge was to get to the right answer before the exchange got too heated. If she got frustrated, answering my questions became impossible. I learned to change the subject so we could both calm down and she could reset. It almost always worked.

Taking into account how my communication and actions impacted her progress was a constant vigil. If I agreed with the doctors or therapist about something she didn't like, she'd see me as taking their side, and she'd resist. Those were moments that set our progress back a little, but eventually she began to see results that were hard for her to deny.

The goal in acute rehab was to begin to jumpstart her ability to conduct activities of daily living or in therapist speak, ADLs. This was to be achieved through all-day physical, occupational, and speech therapy. She was right-handed, and the stroke robbed her of the use of her entire right side. That meant she'd have to relearn to do everything with her left hand and on her left side, which was now her strong side. She had to relearn simple things, like how to put her shirt and pants on. How to brush her hair. How to roll onto her side so she could eventually get herself out of bed. At the same time, she had to do things aimed at restoring function on her right side.

Since our brains are all unique, there were things that happened to Mommy as she recovered that had doctors scratching their heads. For instance, arm mobility is usually restored from the shoulder down. People start lifting their arm before they can bend their elbow. Moving their fingers comes last. With Mommy, it was the opposite. Even before she left the hospital, she could move her fingers ever so slightly. Curious as it was, it was. Any movement, unusual or not, was a reason to celebrate.

I was fortunate that my new career choice gave me the flexibility to be there for her. I visited every day after her therapy sessions. I was there for dinner and sat with her until the end of visiting hours every night. I was there to give her pep talks and applaud every tiny sign of progress. I felt like Fezzik, Andre the Giant's character *The Princess Bride* when he gets excited for Wesley for moving his pinky finger after having been mostly dead all day.

Perhaps in some small part due to my motivation, Mommy always got good reports. The therapists would tell me how determined she was to get better, and they loved working with her. Compared to many of their clients, she was young, charming, and loved to laugh. When I visited her in therapy, I saw mostly much older people who just had a knee and hip replaced, a major cardiac episode, or something else that comes with being a well-advanced senior. In stark contrast, Mommy had a glowing spirit and a beautiful smile that she offered generously. The staff marveled at the fact that she was sixty-eight. During those "She looks so young" conversations, she always sprouted a lopsided grin, smiling even bigger when someone asked if I was her sister.

There was an aide there who she called Taraji P. Henson. He was not a woman but rather a very handsome young man with beautiful dark brown skin and long, perfectly symmetrical braids. He did say, however, that he was an actor who was working as an aide temporarily before moving back to Los Angeles. He looked nothing like Taraji P. Henson, but thanks to her perseveration and aphasia, for me and all her visitors, that was his name. Perhaps it was because she was so charming, but he didn't seem to mind.

During my visits, I entertained and interpreted for her constant stream of visitors. She and I filled out her daily menu requests. I met with her doctors, nurses, therapists, and the social worker to establish and update her care plan. I helped with homework the therapists would leave behind to advance her progress. Each night before I left, I made sure that whatever treats she wanted by her bedside were on the tray and easy for her to reach. I found comfort in this simple routine that ended each night with both of us in a good place.

Holiday traditions were always important to Mommy. Fred and I prepared and brought her Easter brunch. Several visitors came that day, some regulars and some who visited only on that day. We could never have fit into her room. Fortunately, this Easter fell on a warm spring day. Anxious to feel some sun, we all moved out onto the roof-deck with the jungle gym and chatted. Other families had the same idea. Mommy's lifelong friend, Hazel, had been gone a year, but her husband, Eugene, and their two sons came to visit, dressed in their Easter Sunday best. My cousins came too. We sat and talked while watching their daughter play with the children who were there visiting other patients. We had a lovely afternoon. It was as close to old times as our current situation allowed.

Mommy's friend Joylette and I thought puzzles, picture books of places she had traveled, and magazines would exercise her mind and motivate her to get better. But she wasn't interested in reading or even looking at pictures. She was never into puzzles. I tried not to push it, even though I believed it would help with her progress.

Mommy wanted and needed to feel connected to the people she cared about on the outside. That was who she was down to her DNA. I kept her spirits up by cracking jokes and updating her about life outside of rehab. Whenever I spoke about her friends, her face and her posture brightened, and she'd look away from the TV long enough to hear what was going on with them.

Each day, I read her new messages friends and family left on CaringBridge. It was also a boost for me. We both enjoyed the feedback and the online connection. I posted updates on her daily. Her support system subscribed, even though most of them weren't considered the computer generation. They saw an alert each time I posted an update, so their responses were nearly instant. They had become members of my cheer squad, magnifying the praise she so badly needed.

Johnita, her friend from childhood, wrote, "I just read today's journal posting, and all I can say is 'Hooray!' I am so happy for you and all of the progress you have made. Keep up the good work!"

Joylette sent messages often, even though she also visited. One message read, "It was great visiting you the past couple days. From what I had heard before, your progress seems remarkable! As they say, 'What goes around, comes around,' and all those people you have helped over the years are coming back to help and support you on your 'journey.' We will all continue to pray for you, visit, or send you a message here and think very positive thoughts. Keep working with the therapists. They are your friends! ;-)"

The messages friends and family posted were filled with love and inspiration. The narcissist in her responded joyfully to knowing people were thinking about her. That they were rooting for her. That she had not been forgotten.

I never read Mommy what I actually posted because I wasn't sure how much she'd be comfortable with me sharing, even though I believed I was extremely careful about not sharing anything that would embarrass her. My past was filled with stinging reminders that our views of what was appropriate to share and what wasn't were different. My posts were, however, sprinkled with jokes and the sarcasm that I knew the people reading them would find entertaining and amusing, even if it was at Mommy's expense.

I also needed the positive feedback that her friends would insert into side messages for me. Admittedly, the narcissist in me needed the pats on the back reinforcing that I was a good person.

I knew people cared about what I was going through. They asked all the time, and not out of blind habit. I could feel that they genuinely cared. But when they asked about me, my reflex was to deflect all the attention back to Mommy. It seemed unfair that I should express any pain or suffering. I was healthy and sleeping in my own bed every night. Other than the evenings I spent by her side, I was getting back to a more normal life. I told myself that the only troubling thing was what Mommy was going through, and we were dealing with that.

If I allowed myself to wallow in sorrow, to let feelings of anger and frustration rule, then I'd be the one to suffer. I do not like to suffer. I'd repeat "This is going to be a marathon, not a sprint" in my head like a song you just can't shake. It was one way I bolstered my spirit for the long journey.

Mommy's style had always been front and center. She held tightly to her belief that you should never be seen in the same outfit more than once. Her closet at home was bursting with clothes and shoes for every season and occasion. Her well-fitting wardrobe was colorful and sparkly with a healthy dose of animal prints mixed in. Her style was as much a part of her as anything she was born with. But now, her wardrobe was practical rather than stylish. It consisted of pants with elastic waistbands that she could manage pulling up and down and T-shirts large enough to effortlessly glide over her head. No buttons, no zippers, no snaps or hooks. Her "lying around the house alone" clothes were now her everyday wear. Another sign of the tectonic shifts stroke had brought about.

Through it all, I was still working to build my business and be a decent wife to a husband who couldn't understand why I was spending so much time with my mother. Fred and I weren't used to someone else playing such a large role in our lives, so a massive change in perspective was in order. He had only gotten to enjoy me being home when he got home from work for about five months before evenings with Mommy won out.

Part of not having kids meant we didn't experience repeated surprises that allow you to get used to constantly changing directions. No being awakened from a sound sleep by a crying baby or a scared toddler who had a bad dream. No sick kids hijacking our workdays. No rescuing teenagers who had gotten themselves into trouble. We both preferred life without drama. Not that we wouldn't be there for our loved ones in a crisis. We have and always will support our friends and family who are in need. But Mommy's condition represented a long-term commitment that we had fooled ourselves into believing would never come, or at least not this soon. Our calm had now been disrupted for an unknowable length of time.

"Honey," I said one evening after arriving home. "We have a lot of good living stored up. We have travelled, logged many hours enjoying great food and drink, alone and with cherished friends. Other than work, we have few stressors." I needed to help him put our new reality into perspective. I reminded Fred that since we are both conflict avoiders, we were lucky not to be layering Mommy drama on top of other unresolved issues. "I'm convinced we can handle this. Mostly everyone we know is living through much worse."

He seemed to understand. Even if he didn't, he did the best he could not to burden me with his true feelings. At least for now.

Eventually, I got back to my gym routine with my friend and former coworker, Karin, who was a reporter at KYW. She kept me connected to my work family. The gym gave me something to look forward that was all about me two or three times a week. Not about Mommy or Fred. Karin and I blabbed for the entire ninety minutes of cardio and weights. Sometimes about her issues, sometimes about station gossip, and sometimes about my ordeal. Even though it required getting up by 5:00 a.m., I looked forward to it.

I spent my days attending meetings or working in my home office. Each afternoon around four, I'd start powering down my workday and putting myself into my "visit Mommy" frame of mind. Surprisingly, I began to anticipate seeing her, feeling good about the time I was about to spend with my mother. I've tried to figure out why. Endorphins? Excuse to end my workday? I just couldn't (or wouldn't) believe that I was excited about seeing my mother. That's not possible. But in the end, that was it. My primal need to run to my mommy with my problems had kicked in. Instinctually, she was the person who would make everything better, even though she was the cause of my needing to feel better. I still found comfort and reassurance in her presence regardless of how different she was. It was like the way my cat Tortie turned and ran away when I did something she hated, like giving her eardrops or taking away the safety pin she was playing with. Every time, she came right back to me, angry but with nowhere else to turn.

CHAPTER 10

After about four weeks, we had settled into the acute care routine. That's when they told me Mommy was going to be moved to a subacute facility. During her short time in acute care, she had learned to walk about seven or eight steps with two people holding her on either side and someone following in a wheelchair. She was still perseverating pretty badly, but we could see some improvement. Therapy was moving her in the right direction.

Entering into more unknown territory felt like a giant wave was headed right for us. The prospect of new people, new surroundings, new routines, new rules, and new physical spaces was frightening. It always felt like an assault on my life by the people in the facility she was about to leave. They didn't seem to care how these drastic changes affected me. Truth is, they may have cared, but it wasn't their job to coddle me. Medicare was calling the shots, and they had to gently nudge me toward the place the health care system determined was next. It wasn't personal. It was business.

I mustered up the strength to ask for more time. I still had to research subacute facilities. I was so focused on Mommy's day-to-day that I'd done nothing to prepare for the next step. Asking made all the difference in the world. The staff agreed to give me the extra time I needed to make the right next move for me and Mommy. Once the shock began to melt away, I assessed the long list of subacute facilities they provided and visited the ones that came with the highest Medicare recommendations.

Fred worked in the senior living field, albeit far from the actual patient care delivery level. He and my cousin Judy, who also worked in a senior living community, schooled me on what to look for during my visits. Their advice was to visit more than once if possible if you can't visit during shift changes so you can see as many of the people who'd be caring for Mommy as possible. Look for dirt, the smell of urine, stains on carpet in rooms, and common areas.

The acute rehab staff urged me to choose the facility that offered the most therapy measured in hours each day. Medicare's grading system on their website was also extremely helpful. I needed this type of direction, and thankfully, everyone I asked helped me map the unknown.

There was no reason to go with anything but the absolute best. Medicare was pretty generous with its benefits. They would pay for up to one hundred days for residential subacute care. Mommy's Medigap insurance covered the balance if there was one. All she had to do was continue to show progress, and they'd work with her for a full one hundred days.

I selected a lovely facility in Moorestown, New Jersey. It was fairly new, and the décor had the look of a rustic French village. The rooms were painted in warm earth tones. The furniture was oversized and elegantly designed stained wood, like something you'd find in a stately manor. The common areas were charming, with lots of space to enjoy outside her room, which was slightly larger than her acute rehab room, but not much. On the first floor, just as you entered, there was a room with a piano, a living room area with a fireplace, several seating areas, and a quaint French bistro-like space where the permanent residents ate their meals. The movie theater where residents could watch the giant screen TV had theater style seating and plenty of room for wheelchairs.

The Equestrian Overlook on the second floor was something special and really set the facility apart from the others I had visited. This small sitting area had large windows that opened onto the horse farm and riding school next door. This was a place befitting Mommy, the kind of place that would impress her friends. I knew she'd appreciate that.

After I made my choice and got over the shock and dismay of having to transport Mommy to the new facility alone, we prepared for her next stage of recovery. I was anxious and worried, having no faith in my ability to manage this task. She had not been outside the care of medical professionals for well over a month. And now they were entrusting her care to me exclusively. Yes, it was only for a thirty-minute drive, but I was still scared as we entered into new, unknown territory. I think she was too.

After we completed all the paperwork, the nurse's aide on duty helped transfer Mommy from the wheelchair into my car. It wasn't effortless, but it was without incident.

"Does it feel good to be out and about?" I asked. She shook her head to say yes as I drove carefully, like a parent bringing home a newborn. She hadn't moved this fast for a long time, and I didn't want her to get motion sick. I was being overly cautious because she wasn't even prone to motion sickness. She had a cast iron stomach that could stand up to anything.

The route we traveled took us close to her house. I asked if she wanted to drive by, and she again shook her head, signaling yes. It was a brief detour. As we approached the house, I slowed down ever so slightly. She craned her head as we drove toward and away from the house, trying to capture a glimpse of her pre-stroke life while eyeballing her precious jewel to make sure it had not been violated.

The staff had been alerted that we were coming. When we arrived, I pulled into the stone-covered carport lining up the passenger door with a walkway that met up with the main entrance. There were three seating areas along the front and sides of the doorway with comfortable cushioned chairs. One area had a metal picnic table that I imagined was used by residents who chose to entertain their guests outdoors. It was April, so that was a space I could look forward to enjoying with Mommy and her friends when the weather warmed up.

We had moved out of the bland hospital setting, out of the place where necessity rules over creature comforts. We were now in a place people called home. The well-heeled visited their loved ones every Sunday, picked them up for the treat of an outing, and then dropped them back off. It probably did their hearts good to leave Mom, Dad, Grandma, or Grandpa in a place where an interior designer's touch could be felt. In many ways, it felt like being on vacation in a five-star hotel.

I've heard it said that these new stylish senior living facilities are designed for the families and not the residents. If that's true, this chain of facilities had done their market research and built guilt-free monuments to leaving loved ones behind.

A nurse's aide transferred Mommy out of the car and into the waiting wheelchair. We immediately went to her room, where they checked her in and started with all the questions that mark the beginning of any extended stay in a medical facility. Meds? Weight? Height? Birthday? Dentures? Insurance? Living situation, alone or with family? Ultimate goal of rehab?

Whenever I left the room, I'd return to find someone trying to ask her questions and her trying to answer them. Each time, I'd skillfully redirect their attention to me without making her feel like an outsider.

In my painfully honest way, I answered in-take questions that I knew she wouldn't have. We were again at odds. She'd shoot me her increasingly familiar "What you talkin' about, Willis?" look, still refusing to admit she was borderline diabetic. It was as if she wanted to hold on to the pride of not having such a common disease. But she still couldn't say the words it took to relay her little lie. I answered truthfully, not wanting to leave anything to chance. Selfishly, I wanted her to get treated for all that ailed her, minimizing any setbacks. If they needed to treat her for diabetes, that would be one less thing that could derail her progress.

With this new rehab phase, the ultimate goal of getting her home came more sharply into focus. They asked pointed questions about the place she'd go once she finished this stage of therapy. Would she be living alone, or did she live with someone? Were there steps she'd have to navigate? Steps? I'd never thought about how many levels she would have to manage if she went back home. I never considered how getting in and out of the house (something we took for granted) was now a serious obstacle to her living independently.

Her house was once the jewel of the neighborhood, inside and out. Unlike most other houses in this late sixties early seventies planned community, her landscaping was exotic. The other homeowners spruced up what the developer gave them. My parents went well beyond what you could purchase at Sears or Hechingers.

Modeled after the house Ralph and his wife, Gladys, lived in at the time, he and Daddy did their best to recreate the lush oasis of Ralph's beautifully wooded Cherry Hill, New Jersey, community in the middle of Canterbury Green's barren, newly cleared landscape. They had railroad ties and telephone poles trucked in. With the help of dear friends, they were placed with a modern avant-garde eye. Amidst the heavy, dark ties, a white pebble walkway dotted with a slate path snaked through the front yard from the street to oversized brick steps that led to the front door.

The brick steps and front porch were held in place by sand that kept each brick from moving under foot. Over the years, even after being replaced, the brick steps began to shift, creating uneven surfaces. For most people, the unevenness was barely noticeable. But for someone with a shaky gate, keeping your balance can be impossible.

Once inside the foyer, you were greeted with a red, white, and blue tile floor that seemed a bit overpatriotic for an African American family. The design was inspired by the sample house we toured over and over after my parents decided our family was moving from West Philadelphia to Mount Laurel, New Jersey.

The Halifax model was not a traditional split-level home, one where you entered on a landing and traveled up a short flight of stairs to a ranch style layout or down to a basement or family room. In her house, you had to take steps to go just about everywhere. The kitchen, dining room, and living room were on one floor. The family room, office, laundry room, powder room, and entrances to the garage and basement were on another. The master suite, two bedrooms, and bathrooms were on their own level, and a fourth bedroom was up another short flight of steps.

Over the years, Mommy had filled all the space our family of four used to share. She'd have to make a lot of progress to go back home and access all the things her daily life previously required.

At this point, she couldn't walk a straight line on a flat surface without maximum assistance. Yet I not only kept hoping for but was expecting miracles. Expecting that at the end of her time here, she would go home to her five levels and unfriendly terrain. Back to living alone, driving, food shopping, cooking, and hanging with her friends. Without me at her beck and call. This is what going back to normal would look like. I continued to be as supportive and encouraging as I could, because more than anything, that's what I wanted.

My cousin-in-law Diane and her daughter, Jackie, came to visit the first day. They arrived shortly after Mommy was checked in. We all went downstairs and sat in one of the cozy sun-drenched indoor sitting areas, chatting and getting used to the place Paula would spend her next one hundred days. Ralph was there too, cracking jokes with the staff and making sure the transition went well for his Paula. Whenever I'd thank him for being there for us, he always responded the same way. "It's my duty."

CHAPTER 11

Ralph and Mommy's relationship was complicated. It began when I was ten years old, just after our family moved to New Jersey. Mommy had begun exploring the retailers in the area we now called home. My parents were always looking for inspiration and ideas for their West Philly children's clothing store and linen shop.

"You have to see this store in the Moorestown Mall," she excitedly told Daddy a couple of weeks after we had settled into our new house. It was owned by an African American man. In the early seventies, it was rare to find blacks owning stores in predominantly white areas. Daddy's stores were in business districts that sat in the heart of black communities.

The very next Saturday evening, after closing their stores, our family headed home, but our route took us right past the mall. It was seven-ish when we walked into GINZA, a head shop that looked like a combination of Spencer's Gifts and A Shop Called East. The store was a hippy cool headquarters that sold black lights and the posters to go with them, tie-dye t-shirts, exotic trinkets from around the world, and a few items for that underground head crowd.

As we walked in, Daddy quickly spotted the gray-haired, brown-skinned owner. He was tending to customers and ringing up purchases at the cash register. I remember this moment so clearly. It was the kind of bro-mantic drama that marks and seals a pivot point in your life. This story launched an era that I cherish, and even now as I write about it, a warm glow surrounds my heart.

Daddy looked the man in the eye and slowly said two words: "Ralph. Hunter."

Mommy, Lynnette, and I stood watching as a remarkable reunion unfolded.

"Cha-lie. Ruffin." Ralph replied with genuine excitement. The *r* in Charlie was silent when Ralph said it. Ralph was one of the few people who called Daddy Cha-lie. Everyone else, friends and family, called him Bitty, the nickname he had since he was a child. People Daddy worked with would call him Charlie, which is what revealed the distance between them. No one who truly knew Daddy would ever call him Charlie with an "r."

Ralph and Daddy hadn't seen each other since junior high, but they quickly picked up where they left off. After that night and for the decades that followed, our families became inseparable.

Ralph was married to Gladys at the time. She was his second wife, and she had a child of her own, who the ten-year old me considered Ralph's son. Ralph actually had a gaggle of children from his first marriage who I rarely saw.

Daddy and Ralph's friendship was deep and true. Our families traveled together. We went skiing and spent lots of time with them in Long Beach Island, where Ralph owned more stores. The couple's and their friends took annual week-long trips to Jamaica to stay in a villa that, to this little girl, always sounded so magical.

The tentacles from each of our families penetrated deeply into the other's. I have few memories of that time that don't include Uncle Ralphie.

Before reuniting, Ralph and Daddy had both been bitten by the retail bug. The paths that brought them back together were forged by their need to be store owners, entrepreneurs, masters of their own destinies. They were incredibly enterprising men who were passionate about business and shared resources whenever it made sense. After Daddy closed his stores on Sixtieth Street, a once thriving business district that was beginning a downward spiral, Mommy went to work for Ralph, managing a GINZA he had opened in Deptford Mall while Daddy returned to work at the *Philadelphia Inquirer*.

Like devoted brothers, Ralph was always there for Daddy, and Daddy was always there for him. Until December 1, 1995, the night Daddy died.

"Mommy, did you know Uncle Ralphie is here?" Lynnette asked as she looked out the living room window.

Daddy died during the night, so our house began filling with people at around 4:00 a.m. It was still very early when Ralph arrived. The sun had barely risen. He didn't bother to come inside. Instead, he grabbed a rake from the garage and quietly gathered up fall leaves on the front lawn. We could see that he was in a solitary place, trying to process the sudden loss of the closest friend he had ever known. It was as if he needed to keep moving to keep the pain from taking him over. He and Gladys were in the middle of a divorce, so Daddy's death was another crushing blow. During an already difficult time, he had now lost the best friend who was as close as any brother and a source of unconditional support.

A few years after Daddy died, Ralph and Mommy became an item. It was difficult for a lot of people to handle, including me. My father was the most important person in my life, and even though I knew Ralph made Mommy happy, I couldn't come to terms with him replacing Daddy. It's very common for close friends to hook up like that after divorce or death. But in spite of the fact that I was about to marry Fred, the ex-husband of one of my sister's friends, I had trouble accepting Mommy's new arrangement.

I loved Ralph like family. He was the fun uncle. He loved life and loved introducing us to exotic and interesting food and experiences. When Ralph was around, the air was always filled with laughter and so many happy voices. Yet here I was, unable to show that love when it mattered most to Mommy. I couldn't handle the notion that he was trying to step in and complete Daddy's unfinished business. I hadn't let go of Daddy, and I wasn't ready for Mommy to.

I pushed back against all the effort Ralph poured into nurturing our relationship when he and Mommy were dating. I no longer laughed at his jokes. I scoffed at his dinner recommendations. I couldn't even make eye contact with him when we talked. I could only see him through a lens still clouded by the stinging loss of my father. I was rejecting him, treating him badly. I was an adult behaving like a spoiled child who wanted him to stay away from my mommy. I knew it was wrong, but I was powerless to stop it. My behavior came from a place deep within my soul where logic had no sway.

My acting out was fueled by thoughts like, *He's sleeping next to her in the bed Daddy bought? Is he taking over the house that I grew up in? If something happens to Mommy, will he get the things Daddy left behind? Will she want to bury him in the family plot I bought when Daddy died?* I had my own life, and I was grateful that Mommy had someone who she enjoyed. It took the pressure off of me and Lynnette. But I struggled mightily to act like it.

Eventually, Ralph asked Mommy to marry him. He gave her a gorgeous two-carat, art deco engagement ring while they were on a trip to Africa. Ralph was forever the showman. He does nothing small, and their romance was no different. But the engagement didn't last long. Ralph didn't have the stomach for being one of Mommy's immediates. Her lopsided expectations. Her criticism that was never balanced by praise. Her need to be the center of attention on a pedestal lavished with gifts or whatever she set her heart on. Filling Daddy's shoes was harder than Ralph knew.

Ralph loved the big romance but hated the drama. Like Icarus, he had flown too close to the sun. But he was wise enough to turn back before his wings melted. The engagement fizzled. She kept the ring.

Through the lingering fallout of their breakup, my relationship with Ralph changed almost immediately. In my heart and head, but never in my words, I sided with him over Mommy, who was heartbroken by their breakup. The first man she chose to be with decided he didn't want to be with her. The end of this relationship that seemed bulletproof just reinforced my feelings about Mommy. She sent a man who clearly adored her running, not much unlike her own mother. It was an "I told you so" moment, but I knew better than to tell her so.

I felt sympathy for him, assuming that this sweet, funny, caring man had suffered the same way Daddy had throughout their thirty-seven-year marriage. Unlike Daddy, he had no unborn child to bind him to her. No societal dictates shackled them to one another. His freedom was his own, and he made a break for it.

They remained close friends and occasional dinner dance companions. Their long history made their relationship too important to dissolve. Our families were so intertwined that after the breakup, Mommy and Ralph's youngest daughter, Stacey, bought Dixie's. The Delaware card and gift shop that Mommy and Stacey bought from Ralph's late brother was named after his wife. This new venture bound the couple together in new ways. That too eventually imploded, but not without its own fiery end.

Mommy and Ralph were far from done. After Mommy's stroke, he was our A team. He supported me and her in all that we suffered through. No matter how often I asked why he was so loyal to her, he'd simply answer, "It's my duty."

CHAPTER 12

Mommy's first roommate at the subacute facility was Carolyn, a soft-spoken African American lady whose children also barely left her side. Carolyn's daughter moved here temporarily from Connecticut to be with her as she recovered from a mysterious brain episode. Her son also visited from far away, giving Carolyn's daughter a chance to go home to Connecticut to check on her son. Carolyn's children were shaped by some of the same forces I was. Their entire days were spent hanging with their mom. They brought her food and cards, flowers, and gifts. They threw her a birthday party and kept her up-to-date on friends and family.

Before we arrived, they had been through a period where Carolyn was somewhat unresponsive. Like Robert De Niro in the movie *Awakenings*, Carolyn had returned from a far-off consciousness and was experiencing a sudden surge of wellness that stymied everyone. Her children were so grateful to have their mother back, and they refused to take anything for granted.

My mother enjoyed the way their affection for their mother and genuine generosity spilled over into her physical and emotional space. Between their daytime vigil and my evening shift, we had our moms under one or more of our watchful eyes from the beginning to the end of visiting hours.

Their room was a hot spot. It was like the popular girl's college dorm room. Paula and Carolyn had lots of visitors. Carolyn's sweetness and warmth, her children's gregarious personalities, and Paula's charisma drew everyone to them. Staff would pop in on occasion just to socialize. Even people who weren't assigned to treat or look after them that day would stop in to say hi. There were always lots of treats to share with anyone who passed through their room, which seemed to always be filled with laughter.

Mommy's steady stream of visitors began to trail off ever so slightly. The newness of the situation had begun to wear off. My friend Teressa, who had been through a prolonged illness with her mother, warned me this would happen. Once the threat of crisis waned, people would return to their lives, doing the things they used to do with Mommy, but now without her. It's natural, and thanks to Teressa, I knew not to take it personally. It did, however, make my visits more important if I wanted to keep Mommy's spirits up.

I kept encouraging people whenever possible, on the phone, on CaringBridge, and in person, to stop by to visit her. It was good stimulation for her brain, better than passively watching *Dr. Oz* and *Oprah*. I was trying to build the best possible environment for her recovery. It was the first time I'd ever been through this, and I'm really good at things the first time around. At paying close attention to all the little details. Putting systems in place to make sure I don't forget anything. Researching and following through on what I learn. Finding the words and/or the strength to get through the rough patches. She had the best Kyle devoted to her recovery.

I made sure we followed all instructions that were issued by Mommy's doctors and therapists. The physical therapy team got to know me and my daily schedule. They'd provide progress reports and tell me how much they enjoyed working with Mommy because of her beautiful smile and boisterous laugh.

I brought in Julie, my favorite massage therapist, to treat Mommy and learn what I could do between visits to reduce the swelling in her ankles. A few times a week, I would take off Mommy's shoes, get out the body lotion, and massage her ankles, always firmly but gently stroking upward. Julie said that would help the excess fluid make its way up and out of her body. It seemed to work. The swelling went down, and Paula enjoyed getting foot massages. She never turned one down. Who would?

My drive to this facility was shorter than to the hospital and acute rehab. There were fewer turns, highways to cross, lights to wait at during my rush hour trip. No school zones where I needed to be alert while driving through. Those tiny details, getting to and from in less time and with fewer obstacles, probably felt bigger than it actually was. Every time our situation's pull on me scaled back the smallest bit, it was magnified. I felt like such relief, welcomed relief, no matter how minute.

My energy was also boosted by the longer spring days that gave us increasing ways to pass the time. As the weather warmed, we weren't limited to the indoor Equestrian Overlook and the lobby sitting areas. We could go outside and see the horses, cats, and exotic chickens that roamed freely on the grounds. There was even a goat that we couldn't see, but his voice was in the air, and his presence was felt.

In my family, animals always gave us a reason to talk to each other. Joanna shared her extreme affection for all animals with us. She would feed birds and even the squirrels in her West Philly back-yard. It was odd but endearing. She also fed the pit bull next door because she felt he was being neglected.

Before the stroke, whenever I called my mother eagerly, antic-ipating telling her something I knew she wanted to hear, thanks to caller ID, she always knew it was me and would answer the phone with my first and middle name, setting me on edge. Slowly she'd say "Kyle. Dana." Every syllable fully enunciated. Inevitably, I'd respond with a slow, fully enunciated "Mother."

She would take all the joy out of whatever I was going to say and set the tone for the conversation. I'd dryly recite my news, and she'd respond sometimes with surprise and other times with "I knew that already." After we clocked a respectable amount of time on the phone, immediately, the conversation would turn to pets.

I'd ask, "Where's Cody?"

She'd respond, "Here on the bed." Or "I haven't seen him." Then she'd ask, "Where's Bogart?"

Bogart was the cat I got in the marriage. Like Cody, he was also black, but we called him poor man's Cody. Skinny with ratty fur and buck teeth. His fangs hung out over his bottom lip when his mouth was closed. He drooled when he purred.

Bogart loved to talk on the phone. I'd call him to me and put the phone to his little pointy ear. He and Paula would have what seemed like a full-blown conversation. He would meow in response to each of her questions. I never knew what she asked him, but he always had an answer.

We didn't talk about much in my family unless there was some kind of crisis to navigate. But we could always talk to each other about what the animals in our lives were doing. It was a safe place, a loving place, a warm space for communication. Our pets liberated our hearts and gave us a common love.

During my visits, I'd update her about Cody, who unfortunately was not having a good stay at my house. It was an unfamiliar space, and he didn't adjust well to sharing it with our two kittens.

Tortie and Kaylee had not been in the presence of other cats since they came to live with us, and it soon became clear that they didn't like our new visitor. There was lots of hissing, hiding, growling, and urinating on carpets. Eventually, I locked Cody in one of our extra bedrooms, taking away his privilege to roam freely. He didn't seem to mind. He was sixteen years old, and they were flouncy and curious little kittens. The safety and security of a locked door seemed to soothe him. But Tortie and Kaylee were obsessed with the prisoner behind the door. Whenever I'd go into the room to feed him, they'd reach their paws under the door, swiping with anticipation. At what? Only they knew.

Cody was my cat for about a year before he went to live with his grandmother. I got Cody in 1995 to keep my first cat, Darby, company when I was at work twelve hours a day. He was a beautiful, shiny black boy with luxurious fur and a motorboat purr. A few months after Daddy died, I went away on a business trip for a week and left both cats with Mommy. When I got back, I picked up Darby and left Cody behind to keep her company. I figured I'd pick him up in about a week or so. Cats are great company, and I felt that she could use another warm body, no matter how small, in that enormous empty house.

From that point on, Cody only came to visit me when Mommy went away. She had become very attached to him. He was now her cat. She'd fallen for a feline, and she'd fallen hard.

I was grateful for the stable cats outside the facility. They gave us a reason to bond. One looked like Darby, a splotchy Calico who was orange, white, black, and brown tabby. There were black cats and full tabbies. Long hairs, short hairs, friendly, shy, cute, odd-looking. Then there was Chuck or Bill or Frank. I can't actually remember his name. He was a long-haired black cat with a crooked tail and matted fur who spent most of his time at the facility's entrance. Sometimes sleeping in a sunny spot or on one of the cushy chairs just outside the front door. He never actually entered the building, even though the automatic doors would stay open long enough for him to scamper in. He also gave us something else to talk about, especially when he let Mommy pet him on occasion.

The new Mommy exhibited a wide-eyed wonder that I'd never seen before. When she watched the horses and cats, chickens and dogs, she smiled like a child upon seeing such creatures for the first time. Laughing when they did something silly, like when the flock of chickens would suddenly start running to the barn to eat the feed that was just put out. Awww-ing when seven cats would shyly approach us on the wheelchair-friendly path, our perch from which we watched their antics. This new Mommy smiled and laughed more than the old Mommy. She could no longer hold back her feelings. She didn't even have the brainpower to withhold her approval when something I did made her happy. She now expressed pleasure freely. Gone was the guarded, cool customer who measured every reaction, always making sure she was in control of her public image. Sometimes she'd default to her old sarcastic way, but noticeably less.

My mother finally had the relationship she always wanted with her daughter. The stroke gave her that unexpected gift. I now spent every day with her. She loved that I was fully engulfed in her circle of friends. She was like a mother who couldn't wait to show off her daughter in her new Easter outfit. I kept her up to date about them and them up to date about her. I was closer to my mother than I'd ever been. She didn't have to call me to ask with her usual triple dose of sass. "Hello, Kyle. Did you forget how to dial the phone?" Even if she didn't say those words, her attitude when she caught up with me always conveyed that by not making her a priority, I was falling down on the job of being a good daughter.

Being by her side throughout this journey drew me into her life in ways that she had always craved. Even though we were surrounded by her crisis, she had me wrapped around her finger. She sat back while I made sure her life was in order. She wouldn't fall through any cracks. She could do her while I managed the details of her life. In her fantasies, that's what daughters do. Daughters make life easier for Moms. Daughters dote on Moms, bring Moms gifts, and give Moms reasons to brag to their friends. Daughters do the heavy lifting because they're still young, full of energy, and have to pay their dues. I was finally fulfilling her mother-daughter fantasy, and that made her happy.

I wanted her to be happy, but not too happy. She needed to be motivated to get better. If there was anything I knew, it was that a happy Mommy was a lazy Mommy. I knew that because she passed it down to me. Without the tug of fear of failure or of another's expectation, I'd never get off the couch.

I resented that part of myself. Allowing her to get away with it was akin to accepting failure on both our parts. She could have her fantasy for a little while, but I couldn't let it slow or stop her progress. The clock was ticking, and she still had a very long way to go.

CHAPTER 13

Carolyn was discharged about halfway through Mommy's one hundred days. It was a sad day for so many reasons. Sharing the space with her was both comfortable and easy. They came from similar backgrounds, had similar habits, and really liked each other. It hadn't occurred to me that eventually she would leave.

Then the revolving door of roommates began. Roommate roulette always put me on edge. Would the next roommate be a racist? Would they do something that would hurt my mother's feelings? Would they hate that she liked to sleep with the TV on all night? Would her inability to communicate cause a riff? Would they not understand when she was trying to be nice to them? Those questions filled my head every time there was a roommate change, and there were many.

I imagine it's similar to a parent's experience when they send their children off into the world alone. When they go to preschool or kindergarten, from elementary to middle school, then to high school. When they go from high school to college or into the military. Or just out to a friend's house. Right when you've gotten comfortable, a big change comes, and new anxiety strikes. I wondered, like a parent, whether she would be okay, not trusting that she had made it this far in life without me watching over her. The parental instincts I assumed I didn't have up until now kicked in. I worried about her whenever I wasn't with her.

The social component of an extended stay in a facility is ever present. It doesn't exist independently of the situation. It is always a factor. The Ruffins are a family of social over-achievers. Not sure why, but we're all very sensitive about others who are in our sphere of influence. Mommy was genuinely tuned into other people's needs, unless they were immediate family. Pre-stroke, I saw often that she was a natural at making people feel comfortable and good about themselves. But her aphasia opened a door to the unknown, and I had made it my job to protect her, whether I needed to or not. I interpreted for her and performed many of her acts of kindness, the ones that generated a glow in others that came from Mommy showing she cared about them.

Turns out, when I wasn't there, she managed not to get herself killed or beat up. You hear horrible stories on the news and through gossip about seniors being battered in nursing homes. This was not that kind of place, but those stories danced around in the back of my mind. The people there were caring, patient, and they, like the acute rehab team, were moved by her pretty smile and easy laughter.

Every few weeks, I'd get progress reports during our care conferences. It was like parent-teacher night without the grades. Surrounded by her team of speech, occupational, and physical therapists, I'd learn things that were going on during the times I wasn't there. Times when I assumed everything was okay, but if they weren't, care conferences were when I found out. Was she cooperating and making enough progress to continue? Was she eating or sleeping as expected? Was she being a good girl?

No matter how slow they tell you progress will be, it's even slower. And forward progress was often interrupted by small setbacks. Her ankles would swell so badly that her feet hurt too much to do anything. She often felt pain in her arm and would choose not to use it for a day or two.

Every day, I would test her to see if she was improving. She could move her fingers, which their therapists were still stymied by, but eventually, she began to move her lower arm. Then after a couple of weeks, should could lift her elbow off the table. It took several weeks before she could lift her entire arm. Ralph and I congratulated and praised her after each and every milestone. I shared every step of her progress on CaringBridge and with anyone I spoke with on any given day. The messages that followed expanded the celebration beyond me and Ralph and into Mommy's cherished circle of friends.

"She moved her leg!" Ralph exclaimed one day when I arrived. After asking her every day if she could move her leg, one day she did. Ralph, whose regular presence was still a very welcomed source of support, saw it first. I asked her to move her leg for me, and though she tried, she couldn't do it again. After a few weeks, she could move it consistently upon request. The moves were small but oh so important. It meant new pathways in her brain were being created to take over for the ones that were suffocated by the stroke. It meant that her hard work was paying off. It meant that I could continue to hope that someday, she would go home good as new.

Each night, we did her homework. The word association exercises that reestablished relational thinking seemed childish, but as she began to see the benefits of them, she stuck with them. There were pages with pictures of everyday items like a pot or a dog. Mommy would have to say that word out loud. There were sheets that contained names of things that were alike, like George Washington, Abraham Lincoln, and Bill Clinton. Mommy would have to answer with the word "presidents." And I'd mark her answer correct.

In those moments, I was transported back to the time my first-grade teacher sent me home with a weekend assignment to write out the numbers from one to fifty because I was struggling with math. Our entire family spent that Sunday afternoon in Mommy and Daddy's bedroom, she and I lying together on the bed as I labored mightily to complete this simple task. Daddy watched TV as Lynnette, who was in fourth grade at the time, tried to help by whipping through the numbers in a couple of minutes. But I just couldn't get it, and my attention span was that of a flea. It seemed like it took me three hours to get to fifty.

Mommy became eager to complete her homework each night, pointing to it when I arrived, making sure we did what was assigned. I was proud of her and worked to choke out those words as often as I could. She was motivated in a way I had not seen before. Maybe it was all the pats on the back, the continuous positive feedback from therapists and me. Or hearing me tell her visitors over and over how well she was doing, knowing she'd never want to let on-lookers down.

Reading was a struggle, but she was getting better. Her reading voice was improving with each passing week. I think the confidence she began to feel that the right words were coming out helped put more energy into her breath.

She didn't even seem tired after therapy, which is what we were told to expect. They said that patients often just want to go back to their rooms and sleep after a hard day's work. But each day when I arrived, Mommy was wide awake. We hung out together until after visiting hours ended.

Mommy insisted on sleeping in her satin caftans. I brought her several that I found in her bedroom drawer. The fact that she cared how she looked was a great sign. Her caftans represented her old life, a little piece of normalcy that she wanted back. But the colorful floor-length gowns made it difficult to hold on to her when transferring from the wheelchair to the bed. The nurse's aides pleaded with me to get her to wear something else. They tried to convince her to wear something else to bed, but she got tired of hearing it. Rather than suffer through their pleas, she got me to do what she wanted. After two early morning phone calls from nurse's aides letting me know that they dropped her during a transfer, putting her to bed became my job.

Mommy was still skilled at getting what she wanted. She knew I wouldn't fight back, and I had no problem defending that sliver of her old life, even though it created an avoidable safety threat. I wanted her to feel like there was some part of her life she could control. That was a small concession to make.

Managing her bedtime ritual was something I knew I'd have to take on eventually, but not this early. She insisted that I put her to bed every night. That meant taking her for her final trip to the bathroom, washing her up, putting on the slippery caftan, and then making the precarious transfer from her wheelchair to her bed.

With my new duties, my visiting hours got longer. I'd try to get her started well before the announcement that visiting hours were about to end at 8:00 p.m., but sometimes she had guests, or sometimes she just wasn't ready to go to bed. Once she was finally in bed, her water and graham crackers were within reach on the rolling bed table, the channel she wanted to watch was on, her clothes for the next day were set out, and her wheelchair was positioned for an easy middle-of-the-night bathroom trip. I could leave.

I'd stretch over the side of the bed to kiss her forehead and say "I love you, Mommy." Then I'd put my cheek to her lips to make it easy for her to kiss me back. Partly because it was good therapy for the drooping right side of her face, and partly because I wanted to make her feel good by playing into her perfect mother-daughter fantasy.

Saying "I love you" was not a part of who we were. I did love her, but the words had never come easy. Up to that point, I could only remember one time that Mommy said she loved me. When I was in college, I asked to borrow her car on New Year's Eve to drive back to University of Delaware, which was an hour away.

"I love you and want you to be safe. I don't think tonight is a good night for you to travel that far," she said as she rejected my request. From where I stood, she said what she did to manipulate me rather than to express a mother's genuine love for her child.

Mommy's eating habits had changed. She'd become one of those nursing home residents for whom mealtime was the best part of their day. The first time I saw this strange behavior was when Fred and I visited his eighty-four-year-old mother when she was in a nursing home for therapy. As we were leaving, we encountered residents lined up in their wheelchairs and on chairs outside the locked dining room, waiting to be let in. In Fred's line of work, he saw it every day with clients who were well-advanced in years.

Now the anticipation of a meal excited my still youthful mother. Whenever the dinner hour neared, no matter where we were, Mommy would grab my arm, look at my watch, and signal that it was time to go back to her room. She almost always cleaned her plate. It didn't matter that the food wasn't as good as what she was used to when eating out with her friends or the tasty things she cooked for herself at home.

Part of our routine each day was to select her meals for the next day from among two or three choices. She had gotten very good at using her left hand to feed herself, and there was no sign of the perseverated gestures we saw immediately after the stroke. She always found something she'd eat on the limited menu. The serving sizes in senior living or rehab facilities are actual serving size. What you see on a food label is what they serve, not the supersized portions to which we've become accustomed. It never seemed like it was enough food, but she never asked for seconds, so I could only assume she was satisfied. She did lose a little weight, but that wasn't a bad thing. She had it to lose.

One day when I arrived, the physical therapist had left word for me to track her down. She had something she couldn't wait to show me. She and an aide came into Mommy's room and wheeled her out into the hall. They locked the chair in place and helped her stand. They then handed Mommy a cane that had four prongs that fanned out at the bottom for extra stability. With a little assistance, Mommy began walking. They held her by the back of her pants and with a light grip on her arm while she walked several feet.

She concentrated hard as she took her first steps in front of me. Her gaze was focused on the ground in front of her as each foot struggled to get in front of the other. When she sat back down in her wheelchair, she glanced at me out of the side of her eye and smirked as if to say "See? I told you."

I knew that meant Mommy was proud and happy to show off how far she had come. It was such a beautiful moment that I pulled out my phone to video her in action. I played that eighteen-second video for my husband when I got home that night and for everyone who visited for the next week. Each time, she'd grin, shaking her head and taking in the praise.

She was also getting noticeably better at speaking. Aphasia was slowly releasing its grip on her words. Unfortunately, one of the first phrases she got good at saying was "I can't." Before she'd give anything real effort, she'd jump straight to "I can't." She was also quick to say no to anything she was asked.

"Mommy, can you adjust your hat?" That's what we jokingly called her wig. "It looks like it's about to fall off."

"I can't." She was quick to answer.

"Have you tried?"

"No," she'd say sheepishly and then reach for her wig with her left hand, and once I positioned her in front of the bathroom mirror, she'd successfully move it into place.

We were still dealing with the always-confusing yes when she meant no and no when she meant yes. She was getting better at saying what she meant, but not enough to end the frustration.

"You don't seem to be eating the potatoes on your plate," I'd say as I quickly approached to clear her tray. "Do you want them?" She'd try to say "no" as her hand went up to block me from taking them. "Yes."

People who visited often, like her friends Carolyn and Ralph, were patient and understanding. Others were caught off-guard. That was one of many things that compelled me to be there with her every day. I wanted to keep everyone's frustration at a minimum and make sure her friends felt comfortable enough to keep visiting.

During one of my daily tests, I asked her for the phone number of her friend Ernestine. It was a number she had dialed hundreds of times over many, many years. She easily spouted off the correct numbers. Reflexively, she could call up information that she had long ago committed to memory. But when asked to try again, she couldn't do it. Her body and her mind denied her anything she wanted to do, only sometimes allowing her to do the unconscious things she didn't have to think about.

The staff had trained me to do simple transfers. But the most important thing being trained was my patience. I still needed to remind myself that there were new rules of timing and relaxed expectations.

Those reminders came in handy when Mommy tried to release something she was holding with her right hand, but instead she'd grab tighter. Her reflexes were good. If someone threw her a ball, she would catch it, but then she had trouble letting it go. She had difficulty letting go of the wheelchair handle when she was being transferred from the toilet to the wheelchair. She'd hold on so tight to the support bar on the wall that when she dropped her 170 pounds back into the wheelchair, her entire body jerked, her arm's length unable to span the needed distance.

Once in a while, I tried to get her to write her name. She'd start with the "P" and continue writing "P" after "P" after "P." She still perseverated when she wrote. But there was still visible progress where it mattered. When getting her ready for bed, I'd ask her to lift her arms so I could put her gown on. Each night, she would lift her right arm with her left hand a little bit higher to help me. Those small changes gave me hope.

Mommy remained in subacute rehab for nearly the entire one hundred days Medicare allotted. During that time, she met her goal of walking with maximum assistance. Her perseveration lessened. Even though her speech was far from perfect, she could communicate enough to come home with me, comfortable with the notion that her basic needs would be met.

But like before, this transition came before I was ready. They sprung it on me about a week out, and it was a shock to my system. As long as she was in rehab, I could go home. I could keep Mommy's situation and my homelife separate. At home, I could pretend everything was still okay, knowing that she was in the best possible place. I wasn't prepared mentally or emotionally for having her under my roof and being responsible for all the things others were managing for her.

I also had to confront Fred about becoming part of my new reality. He had largely been excused from the day-to-day consequences of Mommy's stroke. This was the day we joked would never come. My mother would never come to live with us, no matter how much she insisted that it was inevitable. But Mommy was about to get her way again.

I was afraid of how the conversation would go. I was afraid Fred would react angrily and force me to find an alternative. Or that he would give me the silent treatment that would be equally effective at making me find other options for Mommy.

"Mommy is being released," I said shyly when I got home that evening. "I asked for an extension, so we have until next week to figure out how to bring her here." I purposely choose words that left no room for options. I didn't ask if. I just made it clear that this was the inevitable next step.

Fred didn't fight me. He didn't resist. He didn't even appear to get angry. Perhaps he knew all along that this was coming.

In that moment, I knew that my husband truly loved me. I knew how much he didn't want this, but he didn't push back or make a difficult situation even more so. The wave came and went, and I continued to swim parallel to the shoreline.

During the extra week, I learned how to transfer Mommy in and out of the car. I ordered a commode, a wheelchair, and a plastic molded brace to hold her dropped foot up. This simple piece of plastic was the only thing that kept her from dragging her right foot, and it would train her ankle to work again. We brought a bed down from a guest room to the living room and moved the living room furniture around to accommodate it. I filled nearly a dozen prescriptions so that she wouldn't miss a single dose. More importantly, I had to jumpstart my mental preparation for becoming her full-time caregiver in the home I had convinced myself that she'd never get to live in.

CHAPTER 14

The transition to my house was the toughest by far. I was now managing Mommy's packed schedule of therapists and nurses who were in and out every day of the week. I became a prisoner in my own home, unable to leave her unattended for more than two hours. That was how long it was between her bathroom breaks, which she still couldn't manage on her own. If I was late, my lovingly chosen red leather chair, the place she sat all day, paid the price.

Twice a week, a home health aide came to bathe and dress her and make her bed. It hardly seemed worth the intrusion, but it was covered by Medicare, so I looked at it as somewhat of a break for me. The other five days, I was the cook and housekeeper, the nurse, the companion, and big sister, watching over her complicated medication schedule and urging her to do the exercises the therapists expected her to do between visits.

She was on Cumadin, which required weekly blood work. Quest Diagnostics was a short drive away, but the distance wasn't the issue. Getting her and her forty-pound wheelchair in and out of my car was the challenge. This was the first time I'd have to transfer my five-foot-nine, 170-pound mother from the car to a wheelchair and back again without help.

The night before our first trip, I felt the stress of knowing I'd have to get her and her wheelchair down my front steps or into the garage. When I came downstairs early that morning, I found her lying wide awake worrying about the same thing.

Fred was home that morning. He helped me get her wheelchair down the two front steps. I pulled the car out of the garage and into the driveway, where there was more room to maneuver. He opened the passenger door wide as I wheeled the chair along the side of my car. As instructed, I locked the wheels and stood in front of her with my back to the open door and helped her stand. We then pivoted, holding each other like partners on the dance floor so she could back into the opening to sit down.

The therapists had reminded me over and over that she should not try to hold on to the door as she lowered herself down. "The door will move, and she needs something steady to hold on to," they warned. The problem with that is the door is the closest and easiest thing to grab when you're feeling unsteady. So naturally, she did just that and pulled the car door in on me. Eventually, she managed to get her hand onto the dashboard and lower herself in. She pulled her left leg in with no problem, and I lifted and put her right leg inside. We both sighed with relief once she was safely in the car. To both our surprise, it went pretty well. But before she would be seated safely again on her throne in my family room, we would have to do it in reverse and then in and out again. We were both painfully aware of that.

Once inside, the woman who avoided doctors for decades readily put out her arm for the phlebotomist. She didn't so much as wince when the needle pierced her smooth brown arm. I watched from the back corner of the room as she exuded the confidence of an experienced soldier no longer afraid to march into battle.

Back to the car, we went and made it through our transfers without incident. This was not the first time and surely not the last time that I'd be reminded of the things we took for granted before the stroke. Popping in and out of the car, walking up curbs and steps, opening doors, and walking through. These simple acts now required advance planning and mental preparedness. I now had to thoroughly think through how we'd get from point A to point B and back again.

After the first trip to Quest, we were told about in-home services, where a phlebotomist would come to my house. I eagerly took advantage of the convenience, but it took away my excuse for getting her out of the house for some fresh air.

I became her handmaid. I now had to add washing and regularly changing her bed linens to my own laundry chores, which already included washing her clothes. I had been washing her clothes every couple of days since acute rehab. The closets and drawers in both facilities didn't hold much. Since I opted out of the laundry service they provided, I had to continually ensure a fresh supply of pants, shirts, panties, bras, socks, and slippery night gowns.

I hid absorbent plastic pads underneath the bed sheets because she didn't think she needed them. I've been in the homes of older relatives or in facilities where urine had seeped into crevasses, making an entire room or facility smell like stale pee. She was sleeping in my living room. I had to take whatever measures I could to protect my furniture, even if it meant lying to her.

For the first time in forty-eight years, I had to prepare three meals a day. She'd gotten used to a meal schedule while in rehab, but I was new at this. Fred and I rarely ate breakfast, and if we did, it was never together except on the weekends. Lunch for me was usually part of a meeting or several quick trips to the fridge to see what would take me the least amount of time to graze on. If I was home, neither of these meals was ever formal, and dinner was usually late. I'd pick up something on my way home from visiting her, or I'd warm up something Fred had prepared and had already eaten his portion.

Her meal routine did give me the structure I needed to navigate this uncharted territory. I like structure. It took some of the uncertainty out of what was expected of me. I didn't have to think about what came next. I knew where I needed to be and when. I didn't have to be reminded or put it on my calendar or experience the jolt of something new and unexpected.

She spent her awake hours between appointments sitting in the red leather throne in my family room, watching Fred's prized TV while I labored away upstairs, managing my business in my office and listening from my workspace perch at the top of the back stairwell. For a day or two, I was afraid to take my eyes off her, so I tried sitting in the family room with her, working while she watched hours upon hours of the Anthony Bourdain and Andrew Zimmer shows on The Travel Channel. She loved courtroom shows, Wendy Williams, and of course, The Doctors, Dr. Oz, and Dr. Phil.

But I spent a lot of time writing, so that meant I needed relative quiet to concentrate. That need drove me upstairs into my office after about a day and a half.

When Fred and I were shopping for our house, my requirements were pretty specific. It had to have four bedrooms even though there were just the two of us. I got into my head that a four-bedroom house had the best resale potential. The house needed a large master bedroom because that was the only bedroom that mattered to us. It needed a large kitchen because Fred, who had been a chef, had an enormous array of kitchen tools and appliances, and I had begun to enjoy cooking. The kitchen needed to connect to a large family room. The kitchen and family rooms were where we knew we'd spend most of our time. Being able to watch our favorite TV shows while working in the kitchen was a must.

I also wanted a house with two separate stairwells. As a child, my sister and I took piano lessons at cousin Juanita's, a relative of Daddy's who lived in (what felt like at the time) a huge, mansion-like three-story, row house in West Philadelphia. It had a grand center hall staircase and a hidden one in the back for servants. It was the coolest thing my seven-year-old eyes had ever seen. When builders started including back staircases in new homes, I absolutely had to have one. I had no idea how this extra staircase would one day benefit Mommy's rehab.

This was the first house Fred and I had bought as a couple. After we put down our deposit, we spent eight nonstop hours one Sunday researching and painstakingly selecting from the builder's options. Fred is an extraordinarily thorough consumer. We carefully picked everything, from the kitchen appliances and cabinets, to the pedestal sink in the powder room, to the outlets in the garage that made installing the automatic garage door openers easier, to the reinforced beams in the kitchen ceiling to hang his pot rack that would hold his cherished collection of All-Clad pots and pans. We even provided the builder with a well-thought-out diagram of exactly where the recessed ceiling lights in the kitchen and family room should be positioned. We were obsessed. Once construction started on the house, we drove over to see it every other day like we were punching a clock. We watched anxiously as our house got closer and closer to becoming our home, fantasizing about the joy of living in it together.

Fred had his eye on a SONY HD TV that was enormous and weighed about 250 pounds. We couldn't find the ideal wall unit for it, so Fred designed one and had it built by a cabinetmaker he knew that builds things for hospital kitchens. Bella, which is what we called the wall unit, was an elaborate place of honor for his beloved TV.

We instantly began decorating, painting, and shopping for things, big and small, to fill our dream house. It was our haven. The space we retreated to after the world had its way with us. We carefully and deliberately chose everything it in. We made a pact that we would only buy things we both loved, ensuring that we both felt bonded to our home. We had moved from the town house I bought when I was single. It was stuffed with my furniture and his from the home he'd owned with his ex-wife and then lived in with his ex-girlfriend. That meant this new house represented and reflected the couple we had become. We loved our house almost as much as we loved each other.

Our family room was extra special. We were big fans of Trading Spaces and devoted hours to watching and getting decorating ideas. We hired a painter who was more of an artist for the wall behind Bella. He specialized in textured painting and designed our wall using elements in the room as inspiration. He drew inspiration from the design on the red leather mirror above the fireplace, the mosaic glass tiles that dotted its slate border, and the artwork we had carefully chosen to display in Bella. He took so long to create this masterpiece that we started calling him Eldon, like the character on Murphy Brown who came to paint her house in the first episode and never seemed to finish. The wall is so exotic that it will probably be the first thing to go when the next owners move in. But we love it so much that we spotlighted it for extra drama.

The space we built was now one of two rooms Mommy the interloper lived in. She had chased Fred away from the place he watched Phillies games. She was an ever-present judge and jury for everything we enjoyed watching. She laughed whenever the Phillies lost and turned her nose up at our favorite science fiction shows.

Even though she had taken over Fred's most cherished space, he never complained to me.

The only time Mommy wasn't in the red leather chair was when she was in bed in the living room, being wheeled to the bathroom, or being walked around the house by Gordon, her kind, patient physical therapist. Gordon and the home aide were both from Bayada, the international company that happens to be headquartered in nearby Moorestown. I find great comfort in giving my business to people I know personally, and I had met the Baiadas. I'd have a place to vent if things didn't go my way. Not only did Gordon, who we already knew, work for Bayada, but so did my dear friend Sylvia. She was a trusted pipeline to people at the top if I needed to throw my weight around.

In addition to physical therapy, the Bayada team continued Mommy's occupational and speech therapy. A nurse and a phlebotomist also came once a week.

Like any manic rule follower who lives in fear of screwing something up, I built systems to ensure that nothing would fall through the cracks. I set alarms on my phone so that I didn't forget Mommy's meds. I put all the schedules of the therapists, nurses, and aides on my business calendar so I knew who was coming when. I created a spreadsheet with all her medications on it. It included real and generic names, dosages, dates prescribed, the doctors who prescribed them, and the last time each was changed and refilled. My pretty little spreadsheet was color coded for morning, midday, and evening so that I could easily tell what she should be taking.

I treated her life like a business, comingling Mommy into the commitments I was making as I continue to build my one-person marketing startup.

Even though Mommy was clearly improving, she hadn't yet regained her ability to communicate complex thoughts. She'd draw you in as she began to tell a story, but it would abruptly end after the second sentence with something like "And that's all I know." It was as if she couldn't keep a thought in her head long enough to complete one of her juicy tales. The situation was compounded by her inability to be discreet and choose her words wisely. Whatever was in her head came out of her mouth without the benefit of being filtered through concern or consideration for the person about whom she was gossiping.

When one of Ralph's sons died, the old Mommy surfaced, and she began calling all her friends to tell them. Wanting to think the best of her, I figured she'd want them to know so they could provide sympathy and support to Ralph. From my office, I could hear her side of each conversation.

"Ralph's son is dead." "Which one?" "The gay one. You know, the one who lived in Florida? He had AIDS."

The call would end shortly after that.

After the third or fourth one, I marched downstairs to defend Ralph and admonish Mommy for seeming to take pleasure in spreading his sad news. But the new Mommy couldn't deliver the news any other way. She couldn't hold back sensitive information, soften her language, or answer clarifying questions. She could only blurt out the facts.

She looked at me with surprise in her eyes and a look that said "Who are you to tell me what I can talk about to my friends?"

"They'd want to know," she explained.

"I know that, but the way you're telling them makes you look bad. Why don't you leave it up to Ralph to tell the people he wants to in the way in wants to?"

After that, the calls stopped. But I felt terrible about how I must have made her feel. The old Mommy would have ignored me and done what she wanted. The person in front of me that day was not the same defensive, defiant woman who raised me. Even though I had won that battle, I was painfully reminded that my strong mother was in yet another way diminished.

By the time Mommy had moved in with me, I was pretty adept at transferring her half-dead weight from wheelchair to bed. Every night, I tucked her in, continuing my routine of kissing her cheek and making her kiss me back. Still telling her I loved her. Saying "I love you" came out easier and easier as her façade began to break down. As I saw how fragile she'd become, I needed her to hear these words as much as I needed to say them. I could only hope she believed me since we never talked about it. Even if I didn't say it, the past few months should have been all the proof she needed.

She didn't sleep through the night. Every night, she had to go to the bathroom at some point. Around 2:00 or 3:00 a.m., the phone on my nightstand would ring, and I'd sleepily drag myself downstairs, transfer her into her wheelchair, and push her to the door of my powder room because the wheelchair was too wide to fit through the door. I'd transfer her to the toilet through the tiny door, wait for her to go, and then do it all again in reverse.

During one of our early attempts, I dropped her, unable to maneuver her weight. But instead of panicking, once we realized she wasn't hurt, we both just laughed. I called out to Fred to help hoist her up off the bathroom floor and position her back in the wheelchair. It never happened again.

Mommy and I both agreed that it was time to upgrade the Razor flip phone that I handed down to her years ago. She insisted on getting an iPhone. She always, always, always wanted the newest technology, but she never, ever, ever wanted to learn how to use it. Her house was littered with "AS SEEN ON TV" gadgets that are always way more complicated than the ads made them look.

Up until this point, I had been paying her phone bill. She wasn't happy when she learned this transition meant she was now going to have to pay her own bill. I didn't need to tell her since she never inquired about or questioned the bills I paid from her account. But I was still operating according to my lifelong need for honest transparency.

The first few days with the new phone were tough. Even if I taught her what to do to call me, she couldn't remember, and she kept calling her friends by mistake. The worst was when she'd call them instead of me for her 3:00 a.m. bathroom trip. Since the living room was just below our bedroom and our double doors opened toward the open living room entrance, sometimes I could hear her apologizing for waking someone up.

I was on the verge of returning the phone for the sake of her dear friends when a friend told me how to use the phone's voice command. Like Mommy, I'm not much for reading instruction manuals. Once I showed her how, she was able to easily use that feature, and now I'd wake up to her saying "Call Kyle Home" just before the phone on my nightstand rang. She used that feature a lot. From my office, I'd hear her bellow out "Call Ralph Cell" or "Call Violet Home," and just as she intended, she'd be connected to the person she wanted to speak to.

We had settled into a comfortable routine, which meant another disruptive wave was forming offshore. I decided to try a new hot yoga place nearby. The class was ninety minutes and well within the two-hour limit. I left the class that evening feeling like I had just had a big personal win. But when I got home, I noticed Mommy was having little body spasms. She didn't want me to call the doctor. She insisted that I take her into the living room to let her lie down.

"That's all I need. I'll be fine."

Selfishly, I complied. I wasn't ready for my yoga-induced calm to be interrupted by another crisis or night in the hospital. Within minutes, the little spasms turned into a full-blown seizure.

Apparently, seizures are not uncommon for stroke victims. Scar tissue forms after the part of the brain impacted by stroke dies, disrupting the ability of the neurons to transmit electrical pulses to muscles.

This was the beginning of another frightening trip down the path of the unknown. Neither of us had experience with people with seizures, so we didn't know what was happening or whether it was something fatal. There would be no just letting her rest, and she quickly came to the same conclusion as her whole body convulsed and jerked.

I called 911, and the paramedics arrived quickly, filling up the remaining space in a living room that was packed with her bed and a full complement of furniture. I stood in the foyer watching as my heart and mind raced with fear that this could be fatal. The paramedics were the first to say it was likely a seizure and gave her Dilantin before whisking her off to the hospital. I was right behind her. I didn't know if the paramedics were right. This new thing, whatever it would turn out to be, was another unwanted surprise in a year of nothing but surprises.

In her tiny emergency room space, the Dilantin was beginning work. The jolts were fewer and fewer, and the fear in her eyes began to dissipate. Then the attendant wheeled in a TV, placed it at the foot of her bed, and turned it on. It was about 9:30 p.m., so the specialist Mommy needed observed and talked to her from what looked like his home office. That was new. Tele-medicine. We looked at each other with surprise, eyebrows raised, marveling at the interesting medical advance.

They admitted her, and after a few days of observation, Mommy came home with more drugs to add to her arsenal. She went from taking nothing before the stroke to taking well over a dozen pills a day. Pills for her arrhythmia, her blood pressure, blood thinners, aspirin, pills for diabetes, and now to control seizures.

After this ordeal, the wave passed, and neither of us drowned.

I slowly began expanding my work footprint, and Fred and I could socialize again. Friends and family would stay with her if I needed to leave home for more than two hours. It was summer, and we began entertaining a lot on our patio. Thanks to Mommy, we were now living like our neighbors with small children, always needing to keep an eye and ear on home. I could now enjoy a glass or two or bottle of wine and still handle the work of putting Mommy to bed.

Once she could manage her own trips to the bathroom, I decided it was okay for me to leave for more than two hours. The first time I did, my cousin Jonathan agreed to stay with her. Ralph had asked me to accompany him to New York City for his taping of an HBO documentary about old Atlantic City that was part of the launch of *Boardwalk Empire*. Ralph had become a well-known collector of African American culture and memorabilia in the Atlantic City area, so he had been tapped for his unique expertise.

The day went without incident. I continued to spread my wings ever so slightly.

CHAPTER 15

Shortly after the stroke, Mommy's close childhood friend had made a grand offer. She would fly in from New Mexico and stay with her while Fred and I took a vacation. At first, I thought it was too big a gesture. I couldn't see imposing like that. But once I warmed up to the idea, I reached out to Mrs. M and accepted her offer.

Fred and I joyfully began planning a trip to Montreal and Quebec. It had become our tradition to attend the Montreal Jazz Festival every other July. Usually we'd drive eight hours up the NY State Thruway, but this year, we decided to fly. Neither of us was up for spending sixteen hours in the car. Mrs. M and I coordinated our schedules. We decided that she and her husband would stay at Mommy's house, which my cousin Jonathan volunteered to clean since it had been sitting empty since March.

Mommy would temporarily go back home for a week the day before we left for Canada. On a typical day before vacation, there are lots of things that need attention. But my pre-trip to-do list was way bigger, thanks to Mommy. I spent the week leading up to our Saturday departure cramming two weeks of client work into one. On Friday, I packed for me, Mommy, and Cody, who would be going home with her. I also had to make sure the neighbors who were going to feed and entertain Tortie and Kaylee had all their instructions. I made sure my house was clean enough so I wouldn't be embarrassed by other people walking through it to find Kaylee, who'd likely be hiding under a bed when they arrived. I rearranged all of Mommy's therapy sessions, making sure they all knew where to find her and what to expect in the new surroundings. I documented all the phone numbers of therapists and Mommy's loyal friends and family in case there was an emergency and we couldn't be reached.

On top of all that, I had to remember to tell Mr. and Mrs. M everything they'd needed to know about caring for Mommy. My head was swirling with details, and my body was in constant motion. With each task completed, a new one would make its way into the worry zone in my mind.

Then came that thing that stops you in your tracks, the wave that catches you off guard. Just when I thought I couldn't add another thing to last-minute preparations on the day she was going home, Mommy managed to clog the only toilet in our house that she could use. Ralph (who came to help get Mommy home) and I plunged over and over, flushing and flushing, but to no avail. This clog was a toilet killer.

Fred wasn't home, so I reached out to my neighbor Al, our neighborhood go-to for everything. He was a retired police officer who did odd jobs for everyone on our block, pretty much on demand. Al dutifully came and assessed the toilet.

"You'll need a new one," he said.

"I've never heard of such a thing. It's just a clog. Why do we need to replace the toilet?"

"This one's not powerful enough to clear itself out." In his extraordinary, just-in-time, helpful way, Al said, "I'll run over to Lowes and buy a toilet and replace this one for you."

"Really? You'd do that for us?" His generosity was staggering.

I instantly said yes. I had no choice. It was the only toilet on the first floor, and she'd undoubtedly have to go again at some point.

Al called me from the store to describe the toilet he recommended. It was larger than the previous one, had more flushing power, and of course, was fairly expensive.

"This thing is so powerful you could flush golf balls down it and it wouldn't clog." Al gloated. "We bought one of these, and it's great." It didn't surprise me that Al had switched out his toilets. The toilets our builder used were weak and slow. Fred and I knew that but had adjusted our bathroom habits accordingly.

I couldn't expect Mommy to know the rules of flushing at our house. She just did what came naturally, but the timing couldn't have been worse. We were approaching Mr. and Mrs. M's arrival, so money was no object. Out of respect for the manly association with such repairs, I called Fred to consult. He agreed that it was urgent. Al bought and replaced our toilet, averting crisis and getting us back on track for vacation.

Within a couple of hours, Mr. and Mrs. M were on my doorstep, ready to take Mommy home. We decided to go out to eat first at the nearby diner. Taking Mommy to the diner felt like a stretch because we hadn't done anything like that yet. But there was a wheelchair ramp, and they sat us at a large round table that easily accommodated her chair. Turns out that the world is pretty equipped to handle such things.

It felt almost like old times. Like there were no obstacles. Mommy was struggling with her speech, but we were all patient with her as she made attempts to be part of the conversation.

I spent the entire time peppering Mr. and Mrs. M with details about what she needed.

"We've moved the bed downstairs so she can live in the family room."

"Here's the schedule of appointments for the week, along with the names and phone numbers of each member of the Bayada team."

"Here's a complete list of Paula's posse and their phone numbers. They all know we're going away and are happy to help if needed."

"She'll need to go to bathroom in the middle of the night, so she'll need to call you."

"Here are all her medications and the schedule for each. Everything has been refilled, so no need to worry about that."

"Here's her list of doctors and the preference about where to take her if something happens."

"No often means yes and vice versa, so you'll have to give her time to calm herself before you get to the real answer."

"I've gone shopping and filled the refrigerator, but here's some extra money if you want to attempt to go out to dinner."

"Here's how the wheelchair opens and closes."

"We've taken an accessible commode to her house and put it in the powder room downstairs."

"Here's Cody's food. He eats in the morning then will likely disappear for the rest of day. His litter box needs cleaning periodically."

"Here's our flight schedule, hotel information, and the dates we're in Montreal and in Quebec, but you'll be able to reach us on our cell phones."

Even once they were safely back at Mommy's, I called again with more information. But of all things, I must have forgot to mention that when Mommy barks orders, she's not being rude. She is struggling to find and speak the words, so she is doing the best she can. This omission is the only thing I can imagine that set off another unfortunate sequence of events.

We flew to Montreal that Saturday. Each day, I called Mommy's cellphone to check in. Our conversations lasted less than a minute because talking was still difficult for her. I didn't, however, call Mrs. M. I should have, but I was just so happy to be away, focusing all my attention on my husband and my marriage for the first time since Mommy's stroke that I didn't take that extra step. Once I knew Mommy was okay, I resumed my vacation without worry or concern.

On Tuesday evening, while walking along St. Laurent Street in Montreal trying to find a place to eat dinner, my phone rang. It was Mrs. M. She asked questions and indicated they were struggling a bit. I stopped on the sidewalk, trying to hear her out while Fred shot me angry looks, paced, and dropped F-bombs, punishing me for the interruption.

She mentioned that they had eaten out, and she took Mommy shopping at Steinmart, one of her favorite stores. I felt a twinge of anxiety because that was stretching the boundaries of what I thought Mommy could handle. But I was also happy that there was a bit of normalcy in their interaction. They weren't afraid of every little thing like I was, so Mr. and Mrs. M did what they thought they'd all enjoy. Things that, in the past, they would have done together.

Fred began to walk away from me briskly. His anger was seeping from every pore, and I found myself again forced to choose between my disabled mother and my husband. Even though I was equally angry at his selfishness, I hastened the end of my call with Mrs. M and caught up with him. On the inside, I was steaming. How dare he behave so childishly? How could he make this even harder for me? How could he be mad at me for taking a call from the person who was caring for my crippled mother? Instead of lashing out at him, I reacted like an abused wife. I tried to smooth things over with him so that we could enjoy the rest of our evening.

I thought about calling back, but I didn't want to risk his wrath again. His behavior was hurtful and stifling. Fred's quick temper was no surprise, and it always shut me down. I never learned how to stand up for myself or call him out on his bad behavior. I was afraid to do anything that might make him react that way again.

The next morning, as we checked out of our hotel to head to Quebec, my phone rang again. Once again it was Mrs. M. "I'm standing out on your mother's front porch with my bags packed. Mr. M and I can't take it anymore. We're leaving."

"I'm sorry. Did you say you're leaving?" I tried to comprehend what was happening as we hustled through the streets of downtown Montreal, rolling my suitcase behind me and trying to find the rental car agency.

"You're leaving? What happened?"

"I can't take it anymore. This was a mistake. The therapist is here now, so we're leaving. We're going back to Philly to stay with my family until our flight home."

My heart was pounding hard. Street sounds mixed with the drumbeat of my pulse beating in my head as I tried to figure out what to do. Fred focused all his attention on getting the car and none on the fact that a crisis was unfolding. He didn't seem to want any part of it. I was clearly on my own. Without words, he was saying to me that his job was to get us to Quebec. It was up to me to deal with what was happening with my mother.

I quickly called the therapist's cell phone. "Kyle, I'm here with her."

Mommy's occupational therapist assured me that she and the social worker would stay with Mommy until we could work something out. "I can't believe her friend would just leave like that," she commiserated.

"I know. But I have a big decision to make. Should I come home?"

"Whatever you decide to do, we'll help you," she answered. "You deserve a vacation, and if you decide to continue on, we'll figure out a way to make this work."

I hung up and immediately began combing through the papers I brought with me for the phone numbers of Paula's posse. I was forced to impose on them a responsibility that I knew was mine. But I also knew it wasn't just about me. It was about Fred. He deserved a real vacation too, and I didn't want to pay the price of robbing him of that. This time, I chose my husband and my marriage over my mother.

As I juggled my phone, I loaded my luggage and myself into the rental car and began calling Mommy's friends one by one. I asked if they'd be willing to take a shift or two staying with her until we flew back home on Saturday. Each one generously said yes in spite of the magnitude of the request. They worked together to ensure that Mommy had complete coverage, never balking at the enormity of what I was asking of them. They also had to be trained on transfers and manage dressing Mommy when the aide wasn't there as well as struggle to understand her words and deeds.

I spent the first hour of our drive to Quebec organizing her friends and coordinating schedules. With each call, I felt the worry subside a little more. I could never repay them for their genuine altruism. The fur lapel pins I bought for each of them in Quebec were mere trinkets, small tokens of the overwhelming appreciation I felt for each of them.

Throughout the rest of the trip, I checked in with every shift change, and thankfully all was okay. One of Mommy's helpers shared that Mrs. M said I never even called her. She was right. Mrs. M blasted me to my poor mother, telling her that her own daughter didn't love or care about her enough to call. I don't think she knew that I spoke with my mother every day. In her state, that's the kind of thing Mommy wouldn't have thought to tell her.

My heart was sick, and I was angry that someone who called herself a friend would leave so abruptly without considering the consequences. I beat myself up for giving into Fred's outburst the first time Mrs. M called. I didn't take the time to understand that a crisis was mounting. I didn't hear her out. If I had, I may have been able to keep her from leaving. It was all my fault. My fault for trusting Mrs. M to handle such a difficult situation. My fault for thinking it was okay to go away. My fault for not realizing that the sometimes, turbulent relationship between Mommy and Mrs. M would rear its ugly head. I wasn't there to smooth things over. I had forgotten to explain the new Mommy to her oldest friend.

On the other hand, Mommy's other friends had been so willing and helpful. I thought Mrs. M would be that and more. She offered to do this. I'd even go as far as saying she insisted. When she made that promise right after Mommy's stroke, she said she wanted to do something meaningful for her best friend. She didn't want to just come visit and leave. She wanted to spend time with Mommy. It would seem that neither of us understood all the dynamics that were in play.

I searched my mind for an explanation. Maybe Mrs. M thought Mommy was capable of doing more for herself. Maybe she was. But Mommy had completely bought into her own helplessness. I had no choice but to play along and to honor her every wish. Mrs. M wasn't bound by the same rules. She could walk away and never have to face the consequences of her actions.

I'll never know what really happened. I sent the obligatory "Thank you" letter and shut that door behind me. As far as I was concerned, that was a relationship that I could easily cast away, so I did.

Mommy and Mrs. M had been friends since they were very little girls, but there were times when it seemed that friendship might be over. She didn't approve of Mommy's relationship with Ralph. Mommy was angry with her because when Mrs. M's brother died, Mommy drove through a raging snowstorm to the funeral, and Mrs. M. never showed up. I only had bits and pieces of what were probably the real stories behind the emotional tension between these long-time friends. But it became apparent that there were deep wounds on both sides, wounds that reopened at the worst possible time.

After our plane landed in Philadelphia that Saturday, Fred dropped me off at Mommy's, and I relieved her friend Carol, who bolted out the door at Olympic speed. I couldn't blame her, but I was surprised that she didn't want to stay and chat.

I took my time gathering up Mommy, Cody, and their things and piled them into Mommy's SUV. She didn't seem at all flustered by all that had happened. That night, we made and ate dinner together as if the turmoil over the last week had never happened.

CHAPTER 16

It didn't take long for Mommy to begin to get too comfortable at my house again. I waited on her hand and foot. Not only did she like it; she expected it. In her mind, she would always be in control of my destiny, regardless of other circumstances in my life, like having a husband. But I had a different script playing out in my head. One that was drafted by Fred, whose livelihood allowed me to ratchet down my career so I could take care of my mother.

Being a somewhat solitary man, Fred wanted his house back. He wanted the space we loved and worked so hard to create together. Our family room was our haven. Our couch was our cradle. His TV was his escape, and it was Phillies season. Then there was Mommy in the middle of it all. She had fallen right back into becoming a fixture in his beloved space, watching his cherished TV from morning 'til night. I knew he'd had enough. He never said the words, but I knew my husband well enough to read his agitated body language and tone when we spoke about my mother.

The therapists, nurse, and phlebotomist returned to their routines, all ringing my doorbell for their scheduled appointments. One afternoon appointment was extraordinarily revealing. I happened to be within earshot of Mommy's conversation with her speech therapist. They were talking about children. The therapist was telling Mommy that she and her husband didn't plan to have any. Then in her best staccato voice, Mommy said, "I never wanted children."

I had never heard her say that before, but there it was. I knew in my heart that this was the absolute truth. Her stroke had acted like a truth serum. She wasn't able to hide her real feelings or keep her decades-old lie going.

Although I felt hurt by what she'd just blurted out, I also found strange comfort in another of my life's puzzle pieces falling into place.

I never fully understood why I didn't want children. I blamed it on personal flaws since everyone else seemed to yearn to pass on their seed. To leave a living legacy that proved they were here. To have someone to teach and to care for. Someone to love unconditionally, hoping for the same in return. Throughout much of my adult life, I expected that, at some point, it would hit me. During my first marriage, my husband desperately wanted children, but I couldn't get on board. I thought I didn't love him enough to share parenting with him. Then I married Fred, who I adore. He didn't want children either. I concluded that we were both flawed. Our wish to remain childless was a genetic fluke.

The day I heard my mother utter these telling words, I knew. I didn't want children because she never wanted me. She never instilled me with the love of being a parent. She never exhibited the kind of all-out commitment to her children that transcends words, actions that silently emit that being a mom is the best thing that anyone could wish for. I was raised in the so-called ideal nuclear family, yet I always felt like a burden to her. I guess it's the kind of burden you might feel if the best of your teenage years dissolved away into the daily riggers of marriage and family. When all you believed you could be vanished slowly, day after day, as you were thrust into something you weren't ready for or interested in. A future you hadn't asked for, yet it was the only future you had. All other possibilities wiped clean, like a sponge to a chalk board, leaving behind the straight line of obligation with little chance of forks in the road that you can choose to take or not.

Lynnette and I weren't gifts. We were her punishment for the reckless act of a teenager. A punishment that would last for the rest of her life.

Sometimes, I'd get a whiff of Mommy's resentment. She would never say it, but her actions indicated that she was jealous of me having choices. If she couldn't have them, why should I? It was like she believed that the way her life rolled out was how everyone's should. We become slaves to our decisions and not masters of them. When I left my first husband and moved back in with Mommy and Daddy, she spent every moment I was home lecturing me about going back to him.

"He's not beating you. No matter what he's doing, you cannot divorce him." It didn't matter that I never should have married him. I went through with the wedding because I'd been talked into it. It didn't matter that two weeks before the big day, I punched him in the face and kicked him out of my car in the pouring rain blocks from his job, in his business suit with no umbrella. I spent that entire day fielding pleas from everyone he could find to call me and talk me out of cancelling the wedding. It didn't matter that a year into our marriage, he came to bed and said, "I should go into the kitchen and get a knife and kill you and then kill myself."

As far as Mommy was concerned, marriage was forever—'til death do you part. She made it clear day after day that marrying him was the choice I made. Mine was like the choice she made to have sex at sixteen, which meant living forever with the consequences. As far as she was concerned, my sacred wedding vows bound me to a life sentence. It didn't matter that I was miserable. My only way out was if he made good on his murder-suicide threat.

In spite of our differing opinions about choice, I pushed on down that straight line of caregiving. I had taken on her position, and there was no choice as far as I could see. Here we were. Tables turned. I never wanted to be in this situation, but now it was the only way I knew to respond to someone I loved who needed me.

Her mother lived to ninety. Joanna was the only barometer I had to measure Paula's life expectancy since we had no access to information about my grandfather's health or longevity. He walked out on my grandmother before Mommy was born. Other than the stroke and resulting complications, I knew Mommy to be extremely healthy, resilient, and stubborn. It was likely she'd be around for a very long time, which meant I'd be caregiving for a very long time. But one morning at the gym, I was reminded by my good friend Karin that there was one important choice I could still make.

Mommy had pulled back on her commitment to therapy. She refused to do her homework unless I insisted. She was becoming more capable, but she wasn't motivated to continue the difficult work of getting better. So in August, I issued an ultimatum.

I sat down on the ottoman in front of her as she slumped down in my red leather chair. I looked her in the eye and said, "On November 1, you are leaving." She looked at me with an expression of sudden shock. "You can either go to a nursing home or you can go home," I continued without giving her a chance to respond. "The choice is yours."

It took a lot of courage and some practice before I could have this talk with the ultimate authoritarian in my world, but it worked. The fire was lit.

From my office upstairs, I began hearing her walk laps around the first floor. She'd go from the family room, through the kitchen, into the dining room, then through the living room, and back into the foyer, where she'd start another lap in the family room. I wish she didn't require my tough love to motivate her. I wanted reason to take hold and self-motivation to be her only driver. But I knew what I knew about my mother. She doesn't respond to kindness and reasoning. She only responds to crisis. Alone in my office, I smiled because every step I heard her take was one step closer to her going home and our house becoming ours again.

Mommy had to achieve certain ADL goals before she could go home. She needed to go from her throne in the family to the bathroom on her own. She would have to go up and down steps by herself. She would have to dress herself and prepare something to eat and then take it back to her chair with no help.

After I threw down the gauntlet, she progressed further and faster. There was still some resistance, but she did just what she needed to do to shut me up and prove I was wrong for thinking she was lazy. She was also afraid that I would make good on my nursing home promise. Mommy was motivated by winning another battle in our lifelong war of wills. Now I had become as calculating as her. I was playing one of her games to get her to do what I wanted. It worked.

One day while working in my office, I turned to find her standing outside my door, looking at me with her "See, I told you I could" grin. This look was so familiar to me. Nothing short of catastrophe could budge her from her comfort zone. It was up to me to get inside her head and push the levers I knew would get her to the place she said she too wanted to be—home. Even though she was comfortable and well-taken care of at my house, what I also knew about my mother was that she'd prefer to be at home, away from my constant reminders about taking meds and therapy homework or scolding her for things she said or did. Home represented independence. I recognized the same chronic procrastinator that I have in me and knew she'd needed a sense of urgency. My ultimatum gave it to her.

As she progressed, we began to venture out more and more. We attended Ralph's big night. The HBO documentary he'd interviewed for would launch the channel's original series *Boardwalk Empire*. There were grand events in Atlantic City during the week of the series premiere, and he invited us to panel a discussion where he and other Atlantic City historians discussed the real Nucky Johnson, and the era in which he reigned.

Mommy wanted to go, and I reluctantly agreed to take her. It was a Sunday, and I had nothing else scheduled, so saying no would have been too selfish. Fred agreed to come with us.

The drive to Caesar's Atlantic City takes a little over an hour. We would have to travel through a large casino with a wheelchair. Not a huge deal since casinos attract an older crowd and know how to accommodate them. But I was more concerned about the unavoidable trip to the bathroom.

Normally Mommy would have been dressed to the nines for an event like this. She'd no doubt run into members of her posse and Ralph's family, who only knew Mommy to be uber stylish at all times. That night, she was wearing her best nylon running pants, a sparkly top, and her grungy walking shoes. We snaked our way through the casino and into a large auditorium and found seats next to spaces for wheelchairs.

Mommy craned her neck, looking around the crowded auditorium for friends. When I saw any, I went to them and let them know Paula was in the house. They were thrilled. Sweet mini reunions filled our time until the panel discussion began.

After the panel, they showed the first episode of the show. For the entire evening, I was acutely aware that we were not going to make it home without a bathroom break. The time came, and I wheeled her into the luxurious ladies room. The engineers who designed this handicapped stall didn't take into account that two adults might need to squeeze into the space. Mommy couldn't get from the chair to the toilet and back without my help. I contorted my body to fit between her, the toilet, and the door, making sure she could reach the bar with her good hand. It was challenging to say the least. But the inevitability of it made any issue I might have had disappear. It's funny how you can lose any fear and inhibition when you feel that you have no choice. You just do it.

After the successful comfort stop, we said our goodbyes and headed back home. Seeing her out and in a place that she would have been had it not been for the stroke was a great victory for both of us.

We began to accept invitations from friends, as long as I could be assured that the terrain was safe or that there was help on the other end. For her birthday, Violet and her sister, Albertha, threw Mommy a surprise party in Delaware. I invited Clairees and her brother, Jimmy. That way, I knew Jimmy would be able to help us get Mommy and her wheelchair up the steps and into the front door. Seeing Clair and Jimmy there was Mommy's first surprise. So many of her dear friends had made the trek.

Mommy held court in the living room, the first room inside the front door, as friend after friend came in to greet her.

It was a sweet reunion for everyone. Mommy joyfully embraced each of them. Michelle, Albertha's daughter, had a gorgeous, spacious home with a door to the powder room that accommodated Mommy's wheelchair. That was a bullet we thankfully dodged. If there had been an accident, everyone would have been gracious and forgiving, but it wasn't something anyone wanted.

Then there was the day her friend Hildebrand picked her up and took her to the hairdresser for the first time since her stroke. I fretted over her going out without me, but the respite was nice. They made it there, went out to lunch (her treat), and returned without incident.

"How did you get her from the sink to the chair?" I asked Juanita, Mommy's friend and hairdresser.

"We put her into one of the rolling seats and moved her from place to place." In my mind, I pictured Mommy starring in a dance scene from a nonexistent seventies musical where people were flung about in beauty shop chairs while others danced around them.

Her progress was evident, and when necessary, I reminded her of the deadline that was set. I made sure to sprinkle in regular doses of encouragement and praise to keep her moving toward our goal.

Mommy had worked hard enough to now rely mostly on the four-pronged cane. She could go to the bathroom on her own and even dress and undress herself. She managed the steps by using the bannister on her strong side, which sometimes meant she had to come down the stairs backward. But she was stable, moving with the stubborn confidence of a person determined to prove me wrong and regain whatever independence she could.

She was proud of herself, and I was genuinely proud of her. Mommy had worked harder than I ever saw her work before and regained enough of her abilities for us to move to the next step. She didn't play by all the rules, but she managed to become independent enough to return home.

On November 1, 2010, nearly eight months after her stroke, Mommy moved back into her multilevel house to once again live alone, and I transitioned into another role. Running two households.

CHAPTER 17

Mommy's speech had improved. It was much better, yet far from perfect. She could dial me using her phone's voice command. She was able to travel up and down steps safely after Ralph installed railings where there were none. The therapists helped her adjust over the first couple of weeks of being back home. We then transitioned to another stage of therapy: outpatient.

I visited her every day at first. I taxied her back and forth to therapy three days a week and to doctor's appointments, and on occasion, we went out socially. I shopped for all her food and prepped meals. She only needed to rely on the microwave, which we discovered was broken the day she moved back home. I still carried the illusion that she'd eventually get back to one hundred percent. But even though she was living somewhat independently, I still carried the burden of driving her progress if I wanted it to continue. My plan was to do so by reintroducing her to the things she once enjoyed.

Mommy loved to shop before the stroke, so on day one, I figured a trip to Best Buy would get us one step closer to her old life. I could have handled this trip easier and quicker by myself, but I wanted her to experience the joy of being out in the world again. I hoisted her and her wheelchair into my car, and we scooted over to the store, where we got some practice navigating a public space. We bought a new microwave that, with its box, barely fit into my back seat.

Mommy also loved to drive and was eager to get back behind the wheel of her Mercedes, so I took her to our favorite supermarket. I was determined to get her to maneuver one of those scooter or cart contraptions. She believed she'd be able to, but she struggled mightily, not always getting forward and backward right or able to stop the scooter before crashing into something or someone. She crashed into several people and nearly knocked over at least two end cap displays and the salad bar. I followed behind her like a parent teaching a child how to ride a bike, greeting glares with a sheepish smile, hoping they'd understand and show us patience.

I had seen parents in this very same store trying to acclimate their autistic children to the world. They'd bring them to the supermarket at a not-so-busy time of the day to help them adapt to the social norms we take for granted. The children screamed and threw tantrums while their caregivers gently stroked them with vocal cues designed to calm and console them. They engaged with onlookers in ways that said, "He isn't just another spoiled brat. My child has special needs, and we need your patience."

It was like that for Mommy and me. Seeing people in carts or wheelchairs at the supermarket isn't unusual. Seeing someone who on the outside looks youthful and vibrant drive a cart into people and displays is something of a shock for people who don't know the whole story. We got more than a few sideway glances. Her malady was invisible, so it was my job to communicate our need for their understanding.

My patience quickly wore thin. After one trip, I gave up hope that she'd ever get behind the wheel of a car and decided it was easier for me to shop for her by myself. If I had stuck with it, maybe she would have gotten better. But I had to pick my battles, and this was one field on which I didn't need to claim victory.

On the days she had therapy, she would get up, wash up, get dressed, and make her way down the eight steps that landed her in front of the kitchen door. Then she'd make her way over to the second set of four steps that led to the family room. Each time I arrived, Mommy was already sitting in a chair in the family room, facing the garage door that she knew I'd enter through. I never knew how long she'd been sitting waiting, but her being early was highly uncharacteristic.

My parents were notorious for being fashionably late to every-thing. Weddings, church services, parties, you name it. Throughout my entire childhood, we were always the last to arrive and the last to leave. I never saw a movie from beginning to end. In the sixties and seventies, theaters played movies over and over without clearing the theater between showings. We'd arrive mid-movie and leave after we recognized the point in the film at which we arrived. Now each time we needed to go anywhere, the new Mommy overcompensated for how much time it would take her to get ready. It was strange that she was now always the one waiting for me.

It was winter and a somewhat snowy one for the Northeast. I was insistent about her not missing therapy, so some days, I'd arrive with plenty of time to shovel any snow that had accumulated and treat any ice that might be in her path. She was deathly afraid of ice, and I couldn't blame her. Each step she took on a good solid surface was slow, labored, and taken with great care. Any obstacles or impediments that might make it harder sent terrors through her. But she had come to accept that I would not let her take a day off. It would take a major snowstorm for me not to show up and take her to therapy.

During her hour-long sessions, I'd spend the time at the nearby Starbucks, squeezing work in wherever I could. Keeping my work flowing was important to me. In spite of giving up on marketing my business, I managed to attract a respectable number of referrals to build websites and manage social media and PR for nonprofits and solopreneurs. I needed to contribute to my household while also managing hers. I needed that for my soul, and fortunately, she was taking up less and less of my time.

Eventually, I cut my visits down to every other day. When I didn't visit, I spoke with Mommy to make sure she was okay. On a few occasions, she didn't pick up the phone or call me back quickly. In a panic, I'd drop whatever I was doing, jump in the car, and rush over to her house in a frenzy, thinking the absolute worst the entire way. Each time, I arrived to find that she had accidentally switched off the ringer.

There was a core group of friends who remained devoted to Mommy and me. They continued to call or visit. If they couldn't raise her on the phone, they'd call me, and I'd get to the bottom of it.

My flexible schedule allowed me to shop for her during the day, which I did about once a week. She'd call me with a list, which tended to be pretty much the same every time. I had done it so often that I arranged her list according to the order of the aisles. But my efforts to be efficient went right out the window.

While I was still in the supermarket, she would call me repeatedly to add something she forgot, something she just saw on TV, or something she forgot that she already told me. Each call sent me angrily ping-ponging from one end of the store to the other, trying to make sure I didn't forget anything.

Mommy spent any time not at therapy lying in bed watching TV. Her bedroom had always been her favorite space, even though she could have spent time anywhere in her fairly sizable home. After Daddy died and before the stroke, that was where I'd always find her when I came to visit. The rest of the house was kept nice only for company.

She had established her own worrisome routine. She'd make one trip downstairs each morning, taking down empty containers from the day before and then preparing an entire day's worth of meals, beverages, and snacks. She placed them all into the colorful canvass bag Ralph gave her and strap it over her body like a messenger bag, and then one step at a time, leading with her good leg, she'd go back up the eight steps to her bedroom, where she remained until the next morning.

At first, I was concerned that she'd get sick from eating yogurt that hadn't been refrigerated for eight hours or from eating a sandwich I'd brought her the day before. But Mommy had a strong constitution, and I had other issues to focus on.

I bought her containers with lids that sealed up tightly at the dollar store, and I gave her a travel coffee cup from my collection of unused logoed swag. She used it to hold hot water for her tea. There was no longer any use for the beautiful place settings, flatware, goblet glasses, and cloth napkins that she coveted before her stroke. Her kitchen cabinets and the breakfront in the dining room were filled with dust-covered dishes, glasses, and several styles of flatware. She now ate all her meals out of cheap plastic containers or containers left over from takeout meals.

Gone were the days of her elegantly setting her kitchen and dining room tables like a furniture store display. The way the kitchen and dining room tables were set the day she had her stroke was how they remained, but the place settings in the kitchen were now sharing the large white table with old mail, cards, or little gifts people brought her or wanted to make sure I saw when I visited.

At first, I would carefully put the food away in the cabinets where they had been stored since I was a child. After a few trips to the store to pick up the same things she requested over and over, I realized she had stopped looking in the cabinets for food. If it wasn't on the counter, it didn't exist for her. I began piling all the canned food and boxes of spaghetti on the counter so she'd know she had them.

Mommy would come down and sit with me in the kitchen while I prepared an entire box of spaghetti and portion it out into the containers with the sauce. I'd cook up a whole pound of bacon and boil several eggs, or make tuna salad and leave them in the refrigerator so that she could access them easily.

When she moved back home, Cody came with her. That meant she'd have somewhat of a companion. Caring for Cody would also ensure that she moved her body in ways that would strengthen and restore her mobility. She would never do this on her own, but she would fulfill her obligations. Each morning when she fed Cody, she would have to bend and balance. Eventually I transferred the duty of cleaning out his litter box to her. The box was in the hallway right outside her bedroom. I moved a chair from the dining room into the upstairs hall, placing it next to the litter box so she could sit while she removed the clumped litter.

Again, we settled into a new routine, and I started spending less and less time with her. I got my visits down to three or four days a week with phone calls in between.

One important task she took on was filling the compartments of her seven-day medicine container. I gave her the color-coded chart I created with all her medicines on it. My business brain concocted this system to simplify and create a process that would ensure nothing fell through the cracks. For me, it was easy to print up the latest chart to take to doctor appointments. I got a kick out of their surprised reactions when I handed each doctor this carefully managed Excel spreadsheet. Even for them, it was a little over the top. But I thought it was foolproof.

Turns out my chart was more about me than her. It was based on my logic and what my brain needed to organize her medications. I failed to see that for Mommy, someone who never had to break down a complex project into its many parts and methodically work toward completion, the chart may as well have been written in Chinese. What I created to make our lives simpler was too hard for her to use. It required more work than she cared to invest at a time when she was simply trying to manage the basics.

On top of that, she took no medications before the stroke, and I was forcing her to be and think of herself as someone she didn't want to be. Someone who now has to manage several dozen pills a week. That was an enormous adjustment, one she refused to accept.

Early on, I'd check during each visit to make sure she had filled her medicine box correctly, and I'd count the pills to make sure she was actually taking them. I set up alerts on her phone that would remind her to take her medicine three times a day, but she'd ignore them. Mommy figured she knew better.

When she knew I was checking, she would take—or make it look like she was taking—all her medicines. Lulled into the false sense that she and I were both on the same page, I stopped monitoring her medicine dispenser. I made the mistake of trusting that she was sticking to the schedule. Turns out she wasn't, and there was a price to be paid.

I wanted to step back from micromanaging every aspect of her life. She seemed to want that too. In different ways, we were working toward the same goal. But it wasn't long before I received a call in the middle of the night.

When the phone rings at 2:00 a.m., it's never good. Sometimes if you're lucky, it's a wrong number. But this night, it was just bad.

When I picked my ringing phone up from my nightstand, her name showed in my caller ID. When I answered, I recognized the sounds on the other end to be human, but there were no words. Curiously, Mommy had been able to voice dial me even though she couldn't talk to me at that moment. All I heard were grunts and clicks and a television in the background. Adrenaline snapped me awake, and my mind immediately filled in the unknown with crazy, scary scenarios.

"I'll be right over, Mommy." I jumped right out of bed, called her neighbor Anthony, gave him Mommy's garage door code, and asked him to please check on her and stay with her until I arrived.

Luckily, he was kind and a night owl, so he quickly obliged. He was also the only healthy husband left among the friends on my childhood street that used to be filled with nuclear families.

I sped over to the house and found him standing beside her, watching her writhe and jolt in her bed. I felt for him. He had just landed in the middle of another one of my family's traumatic situations.

Anthony and his wife, Karen, were not only neighbors, but they also shared many laughter-filled hours with my parents over their long friendship. They were also the first people who greeted me at my parents' front door the night Daddy died. That night, with his arm around me, Anthony walked me upstairs and into my parents' bedroom, where my father laid motionless on the floor. He stood with me as I kneeled and cried, rocking back and forth. "No, no, no, no, no." That was all I could muster.

Now we stood in the very same room helplessly watching Mommy in an apparent full-blown seizure, waiting for the paramedics to arrive. I knew just how fortunate we were once again that my parents had so many wonderful people in their lives. When I called, they answered. I was careful not to take advantage, but sometimes I had no choice but to rely on them.

Anthony stayed until the paramedics came. They treated her seizure and whisked her off to the hospital.

This time, the seizure was so intense that its effects mimicked another stroke. Mommy was in the hospital for several days and then had to return to acute rehab for another round of therapy. For more than a week, they worked to restore the functionality she had before this episode.

CHAPTER 18

I was grateful she didn't have another stroke, but the realization that she wasn't going to cooperate with me or modern medicine was a painful pill to swallow. Mommy had stopped taking her seizure medication because she didn't think she needed it. She had, in her way, told me so when she said she felt fine and didn't want to add Dilantin to the battery of pills she was already taking. I rebuked her and insisted that she needed it. But Mommy was as stubborn as ever and determined to wrestle control of her health back on her own terms.

One particularly torturous and unwinnable argument about her medication—she on one side while me, her friend Hildebrand, and his wife, Gloria, were on the other—took place in her room at the rehab facility. She outright refused to take her medicine. Any medicine. She was taking matters into her own hands. She was going to rely on natural remedies from now on. She used this seizure to try to prove that what the doctors were doing wasn't working, ignoring her role here. Maybe the medicine wouldn't have prevented anything, but from where I stood, it was the only thing that could have. Try as we might, there was no convincing her otherwise.

"Mommy, this isn't just about you. It's about how your actions affect me." She rolled her eyes, sucked her teeth, and gave me a look that I read as not trusting my judgment or anyone else's. It quickly became clear that I couldn't couch my argument in terms of how another setback would affect me. My job, as she saw it, was to carry out any and all her wishes without question. I wasn't allowed to factor myself into the equation.

"I can take cumin instead of all these pills," she said with a struggle.

Gloria, Hildebrand, and I took turns explaining her predicament as logically as we could. We tried to convince her that she was well beyond the reach of natural remedies. Prescription drugs were her only hope for survival, but she dug her heels in and shut us out.

"Bitty would want you to take care of yourself," Gloria said. "And you've worked so hard to get this far. It would be terrible to go backward. We've seen how far you've come."

"Another stroke could be your last stroke," I said, reminding her of what her therapists had told her. "You're smarter than this, Mommy. God has put people with knowledge at your feet, and you owe it to God to honor his gift."

I even dropped the D-bomb. "Ignore the doctors and you *will* die."

Since that didn't work, I had nothing to lose by again pointing to the hardship she was placing on me. Through tears, I explained that if she had a stroke, seizure, or whatever was waiting in the wings, I would have to sacrifice my work to her care. I would have to walk away from building the only resource that would be there to take care of me in my old age—my money. That naturally fell on deaf ears.

Her inability to speak in full sentences or carry out a plausible argument didn't stop her from trying to communicate her feelings. The emotional strain had her so worked up that we also had to decipher through no meant yes and yes meant no. Still, there was no doubt what her position was. She was going back to garlic pills, cumin, fish oil, and hibiscus tea. She couldn't—or wouldn't—make the connection between stopping her seizure medication and having a seizure.

I'm not sure what was worse about this conversation, her stubborn denial or what Hildebrand said to me as we walked to our cars. He'd known me since birth. He sat with my father the day I was born. According to family lore, Daddy was in bed suffering from apparent sympathetic labor pains that subsided the moment I was born.

"You're just like her," he said. He didn't even soften it with a chuckle, so I knew he meant it. Immediately, my emotional temperature shot up. I was not like her. I was everything she wasn't. I was reasonable, rational, and never let my stubbornness become a burden to others.

The real truth is that I am just as stubborn as Mommy. When I was about eleven, our family went to dinner with Ralph and his family after spending the day at his Long Beach Island stores. The restaurant was nice. The kind where special occasions were celebrated. It was late on a Sunday evening and quiet for a Jersey Shore restaurant at that time of year. I usually chose the lobster when we ate there. At eleven, I had already come to love that delicacy. Unfortunately, they were out of lobsters. "Order a hamburger," Mommy insisted.

"No. I want lobster. If they don't have it, then I'm not going to order anything."

Mommy was visibly embarrassed. "People are going to think I'm starving my child to death if you don't order something." The more they pushed, the more I resisted. My anger intensified as each of them tried to talk me out of my folly. I was going to make my fate my own no matter how many adults tried to talk me into something I didn't want. My decision wasn't hurting anyone, not even me.

Ultimately, I won a battle I wasn't intending to wage. The story of that night was told over and over in my family. I'm sure Gloria and Hildebrand had heard it and many other tales that proved how stubborn I am. His words in the parking lot weren't meant to hurt. He had unintentionally stepped on a battlefield mine that was buried beneath his assumption that I was emotionally mature enough to handle the truth. I wasn't.

While Mommy was still in acute rehab, I had the unpleasant task of telling her that Eugene, her best friend Hazel's husband, had died. Hazel died a year or so before Mommy's stroke. They had been friends since childhood. From as long back as I could remember, our families spent Thanksgiving and Christmas together every year until the year after Daddy died.

The news slung Mommy into crisis management mode. Even now, her energy level changed when she was given the gift of a crisis. After I left for the night, she informed the rehab staff that she'd need to be released for a day so she could attend the funeral.

I was furious. I thought it was a horrible idea. In her state, she'd draw attention away from the mourning family. And it meant I'd lose an entire day of work. Mommy ordered me to go to her house and pick up her mink coat. Hazel was even more stylish than Mommy, and Mommy couldn't fathom showing up in less than her best. No matter how much I assured her that I'd go and represent the Ruffins, she insisted that she had to go.

"They wouldn't understand if I didn't come!" she exclaimed.

"Mommy, you're in rehab. They've experienced enough medical problems to know that you getting better is the most important thing. I'll make sure they know you wished you were there."

"I *will* be there. What time are you picking me up?"

It was March and almost sixty degrees on the day of the funeral, so I willfully ignored her request for her full-length fur coat. I brought her something I thought she'd find acceptable to wear, but she still wanted that coat, imploring me to drive by her house to pick it up. Once she stepped outside and felt the day's warmth, she changed her mind.

We drove up the New Jersey Turnpike to Red Bank and to the beautiful white church on a hill. Even though the church was handicapped accessible, I still had to push her up fairly steep inclines. Once inside, I positioned her wheelchair alongside me in the last pew, where we sat for the service, away from everyone in the family whose attention we might draw.

It was a very different scene when Hazel passed a few years before. We sat with the family, and I spoke about her elegant sense of style and how lucky I was that she passed down clothes to me when she finally could admit to herself that she'd never fit into them. Some still with price tags on them. Other relatives of ours attended too since Bennetts were like family, with so many random connections. In addition to Mommy and Hazel's childhood connection, Eugene was from Johnstown, a tiny Pennsylvania steel town nestled in Allegheny Mountains and known for at least two great floods. It's the same town my cousin Jonathan grew up in after his father became the minister at Pleasant Hill Baptist Church. The black community in Johnstown all knew each other, and the church and the parsonage where the Tillys lived were just a few miles away from most of Eugene's family. When we visited the Tillys, there'd be at least one visit to Eugene's extended family.

The repast that followed the funeral was in another room of the church down a long, narrow hallway. Mommy and I navigated the hallway and into the dimly lit banquet space. One by one, people who knew Mommy stopped by our table to attempt a conversation as I translated.

Mommy was in her glory, holding court, laughing, and listening to updates from folks she hadn't seen for years. I watched as she tried to behave normally in spite of her obvious handicaps. There was no keeping her from playing the role of queen. No one seemed to mind but me. In this moment, I couldn't conjure up empathy for her need to feel normal and useful. She saw what she was doing as selfless and supportive. She was fulfilling her role as the committed friend who put her own needs aside to support her best friend's children. I saw it as a selfish attention grab that placed an unnecessary burden on me.

I was blind to my own selfishness and to her selflessness. Hazel and Gene's sons were like Mommy's sons. And my sister and I were the daughters Hazel never had. Their relationship went all the way back to when they were three years old. Their mothers, while walking along their West Philadelphia Street, noticed they were wearing the same snowsuits. That history, with the kind of ups and downs sixty-five-year-long relationships have, was still a factor playing out for Mommy. She would be devoted to her friend's family until the very end.

Following the repast and a trip to the tiny bathroom, one of Hazel's sons helped get her back in the car. We took the ninety-minute trip back down the highway. We were going to arrive after dinner had been served, and her appetite was too hardy to go the night without food. We stopped at Wendy's for her favorite salad and finally returned to her room.

A week later, she was released and returned to her own home. I was expecting at least a brief stay at my house, but the therapy team helped her regain what she had lost to the seizure.

We resumed our routine. Therapy. The occasional trip to the podiatrist to help address her blackening toenails. Shopping. My regular visits to prepare meals, clean up where needed, and check her medications. When I noticed that she hadn't taken them, I reminded her of the consequences, but she was still being selective and hardheaded.

Since she refused to do any of the at-home rehab assignments, I suggested that she at least fold her own laundry. The laundry room was down three flights of steps. I didn't think she could handle getting the clothes down to the washer, so I'd throw in a load when I arrived then transferred it to the dryer. On my next visit, I'd take it up stairs and put it on her bed for her to fold. Every time I came back, the pile was still there, pushed over to one side of the king-size bed, leaving a space for her to lie down. Sometimes, she'd fold it, but she'd never take the few steps to the closet or drawer to put it away.

Some of my biggest battles were yet to come.

"Mommy, you have resources. It's time those resources start taking care of you."

"What do you mean?" she asked.

"I think we should hire a service to come do some of the things I do for you. It's not fair that you can afford the help but you don't want to pay for it. I'd also like to get my cleaning people to come here occasionally to clean up."

She looked at me, sucked her teeth, and rolled her eyes.

"If I'm going to pay someone to clean, I at least want it to be someone I know who needs the money."

"Great. Who do you have in mind?" I asked, thrilled that she didn't just shut me down with an "I'll think about it."

"I'll ask Nikki to come clean."

Nikki, our family friend and Ernestine's oldest daughter. I had known Nikki since she was a little girl, and our families were always close. Ernestine worked for my father in his West Philadelphia children's clothing store in the seventies. Nikki was between jobs, so Mommy wanted to help her out.

She began coming over once every few weeks to clean the bathrooms, bedroom, and kitchen, the only rooms Mommy ever used.

She was also great company for Mommy because Nikki was sweet, patient, and like another daughter. When Nikki was there, I knew I could take a day off.

With that obstacle overcome, I revisited bringing in someone regularly to prepare meals and help with other things. I made an appointment with TLC Homecare at the recommendation of a colleague. The two women who owned the company came by to meet Mommy and assess our needs. They were both gentle, soft-spoken, and full of compliments. It was the perfect sales technique for a sensitive and difficult situation. As they explained all the benefits of hiring them, Mommy sat arms crossed and looking stern like a disciplinarian.

Her only words to them were, "I don't need or want your services. No matter how you explain it, the answer is no."

"But your daughter needs help. You don't want her to wear herself out, do you?" they asked, defending and reinforcing my position.

"I don't care. It's her job to take care of me."

"Please, Mommy," I cried, and I mean literally. "This is too much for me. I need someone to take some of the pressure off."

Burnout is one of those newfangled terms to Mommy's generation. When it comes to family, nothing is too much. You do and do and do until one of you is no longer here. In some circles, dying as a result of the ravages of caregiving is an honorable death, probably one Klingons would equate to dying in battle. Older generations of African Americans will shake their heads and talk about what a shame it is, but in the back of their minds, self-sacrifice is the ultimate way into heaven.

The conversation continued like this for several minutes. The women repeatedly tried to make their case. Our case. Mommy flat-out refused to listen.

When Mommy finally had enough, she slowly and deliberately shifted her angry gaze toward me, and without uttering a word, it was clear the conversation was over.

"I'm done. You ladies can leave now. I won't be using your services. I don't care what my daughter tells you. I'm not changing my mind."

Sobbing, I walked them to the door, apologizing for her rudeness through my tears. I could hear Mommy making her way back into the kitchen where she sat down. I joined her and began to prepare the next round of meals. No more words were spoken.

I had never seen Mommy treat anyone with such nasty disregard. But her anguish wasn't meant for them. It was directed at me. I was shirking the responsibilities she firmly believed were mine. She did it for her mother. I was obligated to do the same for her, no matter the personal cost.

The die had long ago been cast. The immutable laws of black family caregiving were being enforced. I was merely a tool in an old rusty box of tradition. She held steadfastly to that tradition, refusing to give way to anyone I had been influenced by because of exposure to people like my husband and my white friends. People who had outsourced family caregiving by hiring help or putting their parents in a nursing home. Wasting their money on something they're perfectly capable of doing themselves.

She had just schooled me on right and wrong. She was keeping me on the path that had been etched deeply in her mind since before I was born. For now, at least, I was her prisoner, and there was nothing I could do about it.

CHAPTER 19

Mommy continued to make progress in spite of herself. We started venturing out more and more, and her social life slowly started to rebuild itself.

One day, she announced that she was going to New York to see a play with her girlfriends. It was a bold undertaking on their part. I knew I couldn't go, but worrying and keeping her from going would have been counter to everything we both hoped for.

I was glad I didn't stand in her way. The trip went without a hitch. She only took her cane, so that meant someone needed to patiently walk with her through the streets of New York City every step of the way. To the theater, from the theater to the restaurant, and back to the bus. One of her travel companions took the time to make sure Mommy was safe and taken care of. And she was taking the reins of her own life back in ways that surprised even her.

When my cousin Dion, Clairees's brother, got married in Delaware, she wanted to go, and I did too. It had been quite some time since she'd seen most of her family. The Poitiers were the closest Mommy had to brothers and sisters, and they were all going to be together for the first time in a while, many flying in for the occasion. This was the closest we'd get to a family reunion.

The day before the wedding, I helped her pick out something to wear. For this occasion, she wanted to access the part of her wardrobe she had annexed to my sister's bedroom, which was four steps up from her room. She hadn't been in that room since her stroke. The steps were an enormous barrier. But as the old adventurous Mommy began to surface more and more, she became interested in reuniting with things she'd long since ignored.

I walked her up the steps, and as she sat on one of Lynnette's twin beds, I leafed through the extra storage wardrobe she had put in the room because she had completely filled the room's walk-in closet. She decided on a colorful crepe accordion skirt. It was the first skirt she had worn since the stroke. It was usually important to her to keep her brace and dirty sneakers covered, but she was going to a wedding. There was no way she'd go wearing sweatpants and a sweatshirt.

When it was time to come back down the steps, she panicked. There was no railing for her to hold on to. I offered myself as her railing, which I had done so many times before, but this time she froze. Eventually she managed to sit down and scooch herself down one step at a time.

On the day of the wedding, we picked Ralph up at the train station in Cherry Hill and drove to Delaware. Both of my parents had always been great with directions. Mommy took offense at me using my phone GPS to get the wedding venue. She wanted to navigate, and this was a battle I decided not to fight. I followed her directions until it was clear that we were lost. What started out as me wanting to make Mommy feel empowered quickly turned into her sad realization that she no longer had command of another thing that used to come easily to her. We stopped at a convenience store to regroup and for Ralph to get coffee. While he was inside, I plugged the address into my phone, even though she kept insisting that she could get us to our destination. Once Ralph was back in the car, we were on our way. We were lost, but not too far from where we needed to go.

As soon as we arrived and word got out that we were in the parking lot, the men of the family eagerly came to greet us and help get Mommy inside. I took advantage of others tending to her and went off to greet family members I too had missed.

Mommy wanted to walk into the room using her cane, which was a relief for me since that meant I didn't have to take her wheelchair out of my trunk. She was gently escorted to our table at the front of the room, where she sat for most of the evening, except for a requisite trip to the bathroom.

My Aunt Gene and Uncle Jim, the Poitiers parents, had long since passed, so Mommy was the family matriarch. She was given a seat of honor in family photos, everyone surrounding her as they posed while guests snapped pictures with their phones and Dion's friend took the official wedding photos.

We said our farewells and drove back to the train station to drop off Ralph. He kissed her on the cheek, got out of the car, and walked up to the train platform. It was after 10:00 p.m., and Mommy insisted on waiting for the train to come before leaving. I reluctantly agreed.

The train was late. Ralph's encouraged us time and time again to leave. But Mommy needed to see with her own eyes that Ralph safely got on his train. In the passenger seat, she sat on high alert, staring at Ralph as if she was a dog watching for her master. She watched so intensely that it was both humorous and sad. Her upper body, twisted at the waist, turned to entirely to face the passenger side window. Her head was facing away from me, but I imagined that she didn't blink once, fearing that she'd miss something. Her focus was singularly directed at Ralph sitting on the platform.

I knew she loved Ralph. They had a long and complicated relationship. But suddenly, I found myself wondering if she loved Ralph more than she loved Daddy. When they were dating, she left Daddy's pictures up all over the house. Slowly, she'd replace pictures of her and Daddy with pictures of her and Ralph. But after they broke up, Daddy's photos resurfaced. She and Ralph had not been a couple for years. Both had dated others since, but their bond was powerful. Watching him so closely that night was her way of repaying him for all he had done for her. It was small in comparison to the sacrifices he made, but in her mind, her deeds always carried more weight than the deeds of others.

Thirty minutes later, the train to Atlantic City arrived. Mommy watched as Ralph boarded and found a seat. Once the train was on its way, she turned around to face the front of the car and signaled that we could go.

CHAPTER 20

Those immutable laws of black family caregiving can lead people astray. Especially if you mix a cocktail of blind obligation, unquestioning submission to authority, and greed.

This combination can be used to justify things that the law sees differently. They can make a person believe they're doing the right thing when they are actually acting out of selfishness.

The anvil of Mommy's blind obedience was teetering on a precipice over my head. I was yet again about to become the victim of another careless act of omission. The details of a story she mostly kept to herself were about to be revealed. The sins of the mother were about to be heaped upon this child.

It all started the day my cousin Andy called and said he wanted to buy the house he was renting from her. The house had belonged to my father's late Uncle Charlie. After Daddy died, my mother took on the responsibility of looking after Uncle Charlie, a dapper military vet in his eighties who had more than a touch of dementia. My father's brothers and sisters had washed their hands of Uncle Charlie. He was ornery, verbally abusive, and sometimes would brandish his gun if he thought you might pose a threat. Mommy withstood all his anger, craziness, and calls in the middle of the night when his blood relatives had all but abandoned him. She'd throw him birthday parties, and a handful would come. She was the emergency contact the police or hospital called when he acted up or was found walking the streets of West Philadelphia in his underwear.

He lived with his blind sister, Daisy. As children, she and her brother, Abner, were taken in by the great grandparents I never knew. But they were just as much family as my blood great aunts and uncles. In the early 1900s, black people in the deep South didn't bother with

145

formalities like adoption. They just opened their home to children in need, never concerning themselves with legal standing.

While Mommy was taking care of Charlie, Abner died. Charlie asked my mother to take care of Abner's business. She cleaned up Abner's West Philadelphia house, gathered all his financial records, and as she told me at the time, followed Uncle Charlie's orders. She conveniently chose to believe him when he said he was Abner's only heir.

Abner, who had no remaining family, had left a tidy sum. He had worked at the Philadelphia Navy Yard for years, had collected a hefty number of savings bonds, and had a healthy savings account. Mommy had always yearned to be in real estate, and here was her chance. Long ago, she had taken a real estate course, but she never pursued a career. She rented Abner's house out and began collecting rent. While Charlie was alive, that money was presumed his, and she used it to care for him and Daisy.

Eventually, Uncle Charlie died, and Daisy went into a nursing home, but not before Mommy had a will drafted that declared her Charlie's only heir. My father had power of attorney and been designated his heir in Charlie's will, so I didn't challenge her when she said he updated his will designating her. The rest of his family didn't seem to care about him. It made complete sense at the time. And I knew that even if I did have misgivings, challenging her wouldn't get me anywhere.

After Charlie died, she rented his house to my cousin Andy, the very house he was looking to buy. I was thrilled. I hated Mommy's fascination with real estate. I didn't believe she had what it took to be successful. All I saw was another thing I'd be forced to deal with somewhere along the way. I was now at that point along the way. I was solely in control of the pesky little things that lurked in the shadows of the big thing, taking care of Mommy. I was going to make quick work of this, rid us of this distraction, and get on with our lives.

I gathered whatever paperwork I could find in the bedroom Daddy had turned into his office. I took deeds, birth certificates, and bank account information to the estate attorney I had worked with to sort out my grandmother's situation when I sold her house.

That was another tangled mess I took on when no one else would. The house my grandmother lived in was still in her parents' name. They had been dead for decades, and no one bothered to finalize their estates. Mommy tried to convince me not to sell Joanna's house. She wanted to rent it out. I held my ground, knowing that the drug house across the street alone would make it a dodgy enterprise. Even then, I knew I needed to eliminate things that could become a future burden on me.

When I sold the house, the proceeds went to my grandmother and her sister's five children, the Poitiers. Neither my mother nor I was entitled to a dime, even though we did all the work. I didn't do it for the money. I did it so that her family house wouldn't become yet another vacant blighted lot in a struggling community. I couldn't live with that on my conscience. It also would have meant leaving money on the table that, at the time, would do my grandmother some good.

When I visited the lawyer about Uncle Charlie and Uncle Abner, I was whistling a happy tune, expecting to quickly unload this albatross of a house. But as he rifled through the papers, he made telling noises of dismay. By the end of the appointment, I realized I was embroiled in an explosive situation that was not of my making. This shitstorm may have not been my fault, but it was certainly my problem.

I walked back to my car muttering under my breath. "What has Paula gotten me into this time? Why do I have to clean up after her? Why me?" I could have walked away. No one would have been the wiser, but something inside me had to see this through. To do the right thing, I would have to choose between protecting Mommy, who had clearly done something wrong, or siding with my father's family, who would see her as a selfish thief who stole what was rightfully theirs.

To complicate things further, the lawyer pointed out that Mommy had never taken the proper legal steps to control or manage Abner's estate. She had total control of Abner's money, and even though I didn't know the details, I did know that she considered what he left behind part of her nest egg.

I drove straight to her house to confront her. With my full anger intact, I peppered her with questions. "What were you thinking? What did you do with the money? Now I have to deal with this. I'm really pissed that you would do this to me!"

She became flustered and unable to speak. She couldn't get her yeses and nos right. To an outsider, it might have looked as if she was sticking to her convictions. That she didn't do anything wrong. Her lingering aphasia made it hard for her to answer the way she wanted to, and my angry accusations were only making it worse. I knew that, but it didn't matter. I needed to unleash on her. In some way, she needed to pay for creating the mess that lay before me.

After Uncle Charlie died, she continued to collect rent from Uncle Abner's house. She rented it to a cousin who allowed her son to move in. He was brutally murdered in the house following what I presume was a drug deal gone bad. After my cousin moved out, she rented it to family members of her friend Ernestine's ex-husband. They paid rent with money orders until the father died. Then they just stopped. At one point, I thought I'd discovered a bag full money orders under her bathroom sink, but they mysteriously disappeared after I let someone stay in her house when she was living with me. I had no way of tracking them or even knowing if that was something I imagined.

After Mommy's stroke, I continued to collect rent from Andy periodically. Once I learned that selling the house to him would be a long, drawn-out process, the prospect fizzled. I stopped collecting rent, even though I had to pay to repair the front porch after a Philadelphia city inspector showed up at Andy's door. The porch itself was sagging, as was its roof. It was undeniably dangerous. I found someone to fix it and paid with Mommy's money, and thankfully, the city inspector gave it a passing grade.

I worked closely with the attorney to figure out what steps were needed to address Uncle Abner's estate. Charlie wasn't a problem because he left nothing but his house. At least I had a will that would legally make the house hers, and then we could sell it. Or so I thought.

I decided to search Daddy's office for it. I recognized the start of Mommy's many attempts to create an orderly filing system, but none lasted more than a time or two of use. There were file drawers filled with empty folders labeled with what was supposed to be stored within. She only got as far as creating piles that she hoped to some-day get to. Some showed evidence of sorting for a short period while other piles were random. Most of the stacks scattered across the desk and on the floor contained little slips of paper mingled with family photos, paperwork from Uncle Charlie's, Uncle Abner's, my grand-mother's house, and paperwork from her life before and after Daddy died. There were lots of cardboard storage boxes filled with a mix of keepsakes from her grandparents and Uncle Jimmy, Joanna's brother.

I found deeds to houses, birth and death certificates, bank loan papers from my parents' business ventures, mortgage payoff info, and to my surprise, paperwork from a house my mother had flipped in West Philadelphia. She had been secretly living out her real estate mogul dream, and I had no clue. I think she kept it from me because she knew I'd criticize what she was doing. But now that we were in crisis, whatever she had tried to hide from me was coming out.

My sister and I had grown up sheltered from my parents' busi-ness dealings. Their generation didn't believe in telling their children about their financial wranglings, good or bad. I was okay with that. I was comfortable not knowing and believing that my parents had it completely together. I would have loved to continue living that lie. But eventually, I learned about everything, whether I wanted to or not.

For several days, I'd go to Mommy's and sift through boxes and stacks of paper, looking for the will she promised me existed. I turned over every single piece of paper on the desk, on the floor, in the closet, and in every cubby hole and drawer of the armoire she had moved from her bedroom into the office in another attempt to organize. All so familiar. These were the same "One day I'll organize these things" piles that were all over every inch of my grandmother's house. Piles Mommy and I picked through finding cash and strange rambling notes to unidentified people my grandmother thought were stealing from her. These same piles mushroomed out of the floor in Daddy's office, clogging every path, making the goal of finding one single piece of paper seem impossible.

I was growing convinced that there was no will. That she remembered wrong and that I was on a futile quest. Mommy could see I was growing weary and impatient. I'd been searching for days, but she knew in her heart the document we sought was there and began joining me in the office to help.

"Kyle?"

"Yes, Mommy?"

"I'm sorry," she said to me one afternoon as she sat in the kitchen with me as I prepared tuna salad.

Regret was evident on her face. It was hard for her to admit this horrible mistake to me. In her way, she was admitting that she was wrong. That she was careless and took advantage of the situation with Charlie and Abner's homes and money. In our relationship, she was always right, even when she was wrong. I knew this was an admission that rocked her to her soul. She had to confess to me and to herself that what she did was bad, maybe even unforgivable. I don't think she ever considered the possibility that I'd eventually have to clean up her mess. She more likely believed that she'd continue to live a long, healthy life and that the situation would resolve itself. I'd know nothing about her dirty little secret were it not for the stroke.

According to my attorney, Brad, there were several steps I'd need to take to inform my father's family about the situation. I felt comfortable knowing I could trust him to guide me through the right legal processes. Brad drew up the documents that allowed me to manage the estates. I began searching for the contact information of everyone we determined was affected and even had conversations with cousins and relatives I hadn't spoken to in years. I explained what I could and warned them they'd be getting documents from a lawyer that would allow me to resolve this once and for all.

One of those family members was my Uncle Edgar. He was one of my father's two remaining siblings and the self-proclaimed patriarch of the Ruffin family. He would prove to be a really fat and hungry fly in the ointment.

While I was figuring things out, Daisy, Abner and Charlie's sister, passed away. Most of my family, including Mommy and me, didn't know she was still alive. After Charlie died, she had spent years in a nursing home on the outskirts of the city.

I dutifully agreed to pay for some of her funeral expenses. I thought that would begin to help make things right. I went to the funeral and spoke to family members I barely knew, explaining what I could about Abner's estate. I was never good at doling out information on an as-needed basis. I mentioned that Abner had left money and that I was trying to figure out how much and how it would be handled. I explained that they would be receiving legal documents giving me permission to manage Abner's estate. It all seemed innocent. Full transparency felt like the right move at the time. Until I got a frantic call from Uncle Edgar. He told me that members of the family called threatening him and that he was frightened about what they might do.

I've only heard tales about families who get violent over money. I'd never experienced it. Edgar's call sent shock waves through my system. Paranoia gripped me. I couldn't sleep at night. I began to suspect that every stranger I saw was trying to find me to hurt me. Was my safety threatened? And my mother, was she in danger? She was living alone and had no means of escaping someone who might break in to harm her.

I saw bad guys everywhere. Coming home from the gym at seven-thirty in the morning, I looked in my rearview mirror. Behind me was a young African American man in an old dusty car with Pennsylvania plates. My mind raced with reasons he'd be on this isolated South Jersey road. Where could someone like that be going at such an early hour? I could think of no businesses he could be headed to. The light turned, and I made a left. He went straight, but I couldn't calm myself. I was convinced that someone would eventually show up and start trouble.

During my next visit, I made sure Mommy's alarm system signs were prominently displayed in front of her house. I started shopping around for an alarm system for our house. How could I have ended up in this situation when all I wanted to do was make things right?

Shortly after the estate paperwork went out, I started getting calls with questions. And I truly didn't have the answers about how much and when they might see any of the money. Then one day, while my sister-in-law Pat was staying with us, the doorbell rang. I was on the phone and didn't answer it. To be helpful, Pat did.

She came upstairs and into my office with an envelope. It was from another attorney informing me that Edgar had hired an attorney to appoint him the administrator of Abner's estate. I began to suspect that his previous call may have been a ploy to get me to spill some details. That concerned uncle act was a ruse. Rather than work with me, he chose to serve me with papers that would take control of the estate away from me.

Now I was furious and on the defensive. How could I trust that Mommy would be protected if I didn't keep my hand in this? I asked my attorney to respond with a letter stating that I would not relinquish my responsibility and that I would only agree to joint administration of the estate. After lots of written huffs and puffs, his side agreed, but now two attorneys were racking up billable hours since neither of us trusted the other.

I still hadn't found Charlie's will, but I needed to believe, like Mommy, that it existed. One afternoon, as the search continued, I turned my head to the sky and began to pray. I may not be a churchgoer, but I have benefitted from prayer. I can't explain how, but I know it works. "Lynnette, Daddy, and Joanna," I said, "if this will is in this room, please lead me to it."

Then a true miracle happened. My next steps led me to a pile that I was certain I had gone through before. It was there that I found it. Charlie's will inside an envelope with several copies. I finally had one little victory.

I drove home and quickly faxed it over to Brad, who immediately called me. "Charlie's signature is not on this will. Even though it was notarized with witnesses and all, there is no space for him to even sign."

I couldn't believe what I was hearing. What kind of rinky-dink lawyer did my mother have draft this will? Who wouldn't include a signature line for the person whose will it was? What a complete disaster.

I continued back and forth with my attorney as he helped us transfer what remained in Uncle Abner's bank account to an estate account, removing Mommy's name and her ability to access the money. This required a trip into Philadelphia, pushing Mommy through the downtown streets. She hadn't been into the city since the stroke.

We started out at Brad's Center City office. In a conference room, they began trying to get answers to what had happened to the one hundred thousand dollars in savings bonds that we could find no trace of.

"Do you recall the total value of the bonds?" Brad asked.

"Yes. No," Mommy said as her head circled around, trying to sync with her response.

"Do you remember spending the money?" he continued.

"No. I mean yes."

"Is it yes or no, Mommy?" I tried to get a definite answer. "Did you deposit that money in the bank?"

"No," she responded.

"So you spent it?" I asked.

"I don't remember."

Having gotten what we could out of her, which was nothing at all, we rolled down the uneven sidewalks and streets of Philadelphia to the bank to take her name off the account and relinquish control to our attorney and Uncle Edgar's.

We could never find a trail. We assumed that she had put them into the bank account and over time spent the money. The attorneys took over from there, negotiating how Mommy would repay what she'd spent. They drafted documents that, as her power of attorney, I signed on her behalf. Then they began a forensic accounting investigation to determine all she owed.

CHAPTER 21

We again settled back into our routines. Mommy's outpatient therapy sessions were coming to an end. Medicare pays for ninety days of therapy, and she had exhausted her allotment. I still managed her homelife while she laid in bed watching TV.

"I feel myself getting stronger," she declared one day after a therapy session. I saw this as an opportunity to get her to use the collapsible walker that I had gotten her. It had wheels and a seat, and it was much lighter than the wheelchair. She refused. Partly because she couldn't flex her right ankle, the one that had been affected by the stroke. She also hated the brace she had to wear to keep her foot at a ninety-degree angle. Even with it, her foot dragged behind her. To compensate, she had to lift and swing her foot around to move forward. Each time she tried, her foot would hit the wheel of the walker, making it hard for her to keep her balance. Fighting for her independence and mine, I kept pushing, insisting, threatening.

The battle of wills reached its ultimate intensity when I forced her to walk outside her house with the walker. "I'm not doing this for me, Mommy. I'm doing this so that you can get back to your old life."

Reluctantly, she came outside and walked clumsily down the driveway to the sidewalk, her ability to balance challenged again and again. Her frustration built up and quickly turned to anger. The fifty feet of sidewalk that I insisted she attempt wasn't perfect. The roots of the old trees at the curb had lifted the cement in places, making it difficult for her to trust her next step.

That was what she'd encounter in the world that we both wanted her to return to. Uneven, unpredictable landscapes that she needed to relearn how to navigate. Her tendency was to walk looking down at where her foot and cane would land next. At the therapist's urging, I tried desperately to teach her to look further ahead so she could prepare herself for what lay before her. She'd try it a few times but quickly revert back to walking in ways that threatened her stability.

Fueled by frustration, we both flared up. I wanted her to continue to get better, and she was resisting what I knew was best. She didn't want to fall. She just wanted to be safely back in her bedroom.

In a fit of rage, I jumped in my car, leaving her stranded on the sidewalk with nothing to get her back into the house but the walker. I pulled away, watching her in my rearview mirror as she struggled.

In spite of what I convinced myself was tough love, I would not have been able to live with myself if something had happened to her because I got angry. I circled the block, returning to find the garage door closed. Seeing that, I knew she was safely back into the house. I drove home, still stewing in my own juices, and went about my day.

Tough love, if that's what it was, failed that day. She never tried to use that walker again. Even though in most cases, she could walk moderate distances with the cane, I always had to bring the huge and heavy wheelchair to bridge the distance between how far she could walk and how far we had to go.

It was around that time I had the sudden realization that I was in mourning. It hit me while I was driving that familiar route to her house. Like a bolt of lightning, I instantly understood that my mother, the woman I knew all my life, was gone. She wasn't dead, but the person she used to be was.

Even though we had our issues, she was still my mother. She was the human being I had known longer than any other. One of two people I could count on if I was in a real crisis. And if Fred were to leave me, Mommy would take me in. Mommy was my lifelong safety net and the last remaining member of a family unit that I found comfort in and understood how to be part of. But our old relationship was over, and I was still playing by its rules. I was struggling upstream to get to a place that we'd never be again.

She would never again be the stylish woman who loved to travel. The person who they invented cellphones for because she was never home. The attentive friend to all the people she cared about.

The person whose words and actions I had come to terms with and knew how to navigate. That Mommy was gone forever.

I understood in that moment that I had to let go of who she was and deal with who she had become. She'll never want to dress the way she used to or go out the way she did. She'd never even talk the way she used to, and I needed to be okay with that. This was our new reality, our new normal. Instead of feeling sad, this realization brought great relief. I felt tension leave my body immediately.

Holding on to the past was a huge burden that I had put on myself. Even if she completely recovered every single thing she lost with the stroke, our relationship would never be the same. I would always be worried that it might happen again. I would always be concerned about her health and well-being. The reality was that we would never go back to those days when we rarely spoke, and I was blindly confident that she was safe.

I attended a stroke caregiver's workshop at a women's conference where I was speaking later in the day about small business marketing. A nurse shared a story about a couple she worked with. The husband had suffered a debilitating stroke and was home in his wife's care. Every day, the wife would dress him in his finest even if they weren't leaving the house. "That's how he always dressed," the wife told the nurse. "I'm just doing what he wants."

It turned out that the husband hated getting dressed up every day. The stroke had robbed him of his flashy side. He just wanted to be comfortable, but she wanted her old husband back.

That's where the letting go is such a relief. The wife was holding on to a husband she'd never have again while reluctantly tending to the person he had become. Dressing a man with limited functionality who was bound to a wheelchair in slacks, a button-down shirt, tie, and jacket is extremely hard work. It can be hard to see that surrendering to elastic waistbands and pullover tops is not the end. It's not giving up. It's accepting the new phase in a long relationship. Sometimes it's good enough to make sure they're not naked.

Just like the wife, I had been holding onto two realities. I was dealing every day with the burdens of stroke while working on a goal of getting Mommy and our relationship to a place she and I would never be again. I refused to accept the person stroke had turned her into and continued pushing us toward the impossible. Carrying the weight of both realities was making this journey harder than it needed to be.

I wonder if my new acceptance turned off my fight. While there was still plenty of internal struggle for me to deal with, was I giving up on being her cheerleader, the person who would push her beyond the limits she set for herself? Would I no longer try to make her see that there were rewards to hard work? Or was I running out of steam? Maybe I was cooperating with the inevitable, pacing myself for the many challenges that were still ahead for an unknowable amount of time.

CHAPTER 22

The big waves, the ones that look like they'll overtake us, are not the only places trouble lies. It can also hide in the shallow water near the shore. When you think you've figured it out and you're close enough to the shoreline to be safe, the undertow can drop you to your knees and take you under with little warning.

Over the next few months, there were lots of times when I thought I was in control and that we were headed in a good direction. Like when Mommy's cardiologist convinced us that there was a procedure that might be able to shock her heart back into a sinus rhythm. That's how a regular heart beats. A-fib meant Mommy's heart stuttered and stammered, allowing blood to pool in front of the heart valve, where it could clot and lead to another stroke.

We took several trips to the heart and lung center in Browns Mills, New Jersey. The hospital was about a thirty-minute drive from my house, but in the opposite direction of Mommy's house. Each appointment meant at least a half-day away from my office, but I did it because both of us saw this as an opportunity to reduce the number of pills she was and wasn't taking. On the day of the procedure, we spent the full day in the hospital starting at 7:00 a.m. I picked Mommy up at 6:00 a.m. for the forty-five-minute drive. The only good part of the day was that Clairees and Ralph spent it with me. I was happy to have their company.

After the procedure, I craftily got them to keep her overnight for observation so that I could get a little break. Otherwise, she would have been at my house, which was something from which I needed to spare Fred.

During one of the follow-up appointments, we were told it didn't work. That was the day her cardiologist callously scolded me for complaining about coming all the way out there.

"I come out here every day," he said. "It's not that far." He seemed to forget that he was being paid to drive the distance and probably pretty handsomely. My business income was determined by billable hours, which meant I was losing money with every trip.

We spent Easter in the ER. I had stopped by to bring food and Easter flowers. Through the years, Mommy made it clear that Easter flowers were as much an obligation as a birthday or Christmas present. Dutifully, I obliged. When I arrived, she said she wasn't feeling well. She even said yes when I asked her if she wanted to go to the hospital.

We spent the entire day and well into the evening in a tiny curtained off room in the ER. Tests indicated that she was primed for another seizure. That happened at least one more day when I came to visit, and we ended up spending the entire afternoon in the ER.

She had reached a place medically where she needed to take absolutely everything prescribed for her, but she believed otherwise. These brief hospital trips did nothing to convince her that her seizure medication was not optional. These minor episodes with outcomes that weren't as catastrophic as previous ones seem to prove her point that her self-prescribed course was fine.

I gave in and became less vigilant about checking her medications. Even though she had a history and an inclination toward noncompliance, she had lulled me into the false sense that she was cooperating. Periodic checks of her medicine container bore that out, but she played me. Once she knew I stopped checking, she started skipping pills she didn't like. During one spot check of her meds, I saw evidence that she had stopped taking her blood thinner. With a condition like hers, I couldn't accept this.

"I noticed bruising on my leg," she told me. "That's why I didn't want to take it."

When I went home that night, I looked up the side effects. Bruising was possible, but it was not a recommended reason to stop taking the medication. I reported that to her, and she said she'd start taking it again.

In the meantime, Fred and I were planning a dream vacation to Ireland and Scotland. It had been over a year since the Montreal catastrophe, and we'd been experimenting with shorter trips. We spent a long weekend in Washington, DC, over the Christmas holidays, and Mommy was fine. We now felt good about taking the leap into a grand adventure by going somewhere we'd never been. We were planning the trip with our good friends Matt and Marci and members of their family.

Even planning the trip was fun. We talked about it for months, preparing for unknown adventures in a land I've only seen in pictures. Fred and I were going to travel to Ireland for a few days with Marci's daughter and her boyfriend. Then we'd all meet up in Edinburgh, Scotland, to drive across the country to the tiny town of Oban. They had taken similar trips, traveling from one single malt Scotch distillery to another. We tasted what they brought back and loved the idea of seeing these places for ourselves.

Because it was such a big trip, when Fred asked if he should buy travel insurance, which we never, ever do, I said yes.

"Why?" he asked.

"Please just get it."

Since going away always meant prepping two households, about a week before the trip, I got busy filling prescriptions, shopping for food, and making sure all her friends knew how to reach me in case of an emergency. We were going to be gone about eleven days, which was a long time for us. But everything was good. We were in those safe, shallow waters where nothing could possibly happen. She was having a good run, and we could go do us.

The day we were to depart, I realized I forgot to take my itinerary over to Mommy's when I brought the last round of groceries the day before. Whenever either of us traveled, we shared our official itinerary with the other. Flight times and numbers, hotel names, addresses, and phone numbers. It comforted us to know that family knew where we were. It had come in particularly handy when Mommy was traveling in Peru and there was a major earthquake in the region. I spent my entire day trying to track her according to her itinerary. I eventually caught up with her group and confirmed they were okay.

I had emailed my Ireland-Scotland itinerary to everyone else, but she needed a hard copy. After I finished packing, I jumped in the car for a quick trip to take it over to her. We hadn't spoken since the day before. When I got to her house, I called out for her from downstairs, but she didn't answer.

I went upstairs into her bedroom, continuing to call her. She still didn't answer. The TV was on, so I knew she was up. I walked over to the bathroom door of her master suite. It was ajar, and I could see her sitting on the toilet. As I opened the door, she looked up at me and reached out her hand. She tried to speak, but no words or sounds came out.

I immediately pulled out my phone and called 911. Then I called Fred.

"You won't believe this," I said. "I think my mother is having another stroke. I've just called 911. The doorbell just rang, so I think they're here. I'll call you back."

We were supposed to leave for the airport in an hour. I was just checking the last thing off my list. And now this.

Once she was safely on her way in the ambulance, I called Fred back and insisted that he go without me. "There's no reason both of us has to stay home."

"No," he said. "I don't want to go without you."

"I'd rather you be there than hovering over me here. There's really nothing you can do here. Maybe I'll still be able to come later."

"No," he said. "I'm staying here with you."

"Please reconsider. But for now, I have to get to the hospital."

As I drove to the hospital, Fred called and said, "I've unpacked and repacked our suitcases, and I'm going. Hopefully you can meet us there later."

I was relieved. I didn't want to have to manage his disappointment when I really needed to focus on Mommy. I had traveled this road by myself, mostly without his help, so I didn't need him to lean on. I had other people for that. I had Ralph and Clairees. They had become my support system in ways I couldn't have imagined.

Fred headed to the airport as I head to the all-too-familiar ER to answer questions, make decisions, and place important calls. The doctors determined that Mommy needed to go to a regional stroke center. The closest one was in Trenton. I wanted the best for Mommy, so I tried to push away the feelings of disappointment that she'd be at a hospital over thirty miles away. Each visit meant close to an hour drive in each direction.

Like the first stroke, I couldn't tell how long it had been. The local doctors decided that the experts in Trenton should determine whether to give her t-PA, the blood thinner that can reduce the damaging effects from stroke.

Mommy had remained conscious from the time I arrived at her house all the way through the ambulance rides and then as they admitted her into the cardiac ICU. Like the first time, she just kept asking "What happened?" Clair and my cousin Judy had joined us in Trenton. We'd take turns telling her that she had another stroke, placating her for a few minutes before she'd ask again.

The doctors determined that it was too late for t-PA. They sat me down to tell me how they thought things might progress from here. Aphasia had already begun to set in, so she may or may not have been repeatedly asking what happened intentionally.

The doctor confirmed that this was a bigger stroke than the first one. "Typically, what we see with strokes like this is that the brain will swell to a dangerous point. We will do everything we can over the next seventy-two hours to keep swelling to a minimum, but we're just not sure how she'll respond."

The unspoken message running beneath this conversation was that this stroke could be fatal. It was so big that the swelling might press against her skull to the point where she'd become brain dead. Even though she was still conscious and speaking, doctors warned that would change if swelling began.

Within a couple of hours, Mommy began to get visibly tired. She no longer asked what happened. She just got drowsier and drowsier. This, they said, was one of the signs that her brain was becoming enlarged.

We parked ourselves in her room, leaving only when the nurses asked us to. I took one of those opportunities to call her friend Ernestine. I needed to tell her what was happening. Once I heard the words come out of my mouth that Mommy might not make it, I began to weep.

As the enormity of our situation came down on me, my weeps turned into full-blown crying. I paced around the parking lot, crying uncontrollably. This could very well be the end. Mommy was about to die. Although I knew I had done everything I could for her and caring for her was a major burden, I wasn't ready for this. I wasn't ready to lose her entirely. The more I thought about it, the harder I cried. And here I was, without Fred, dealing with what could be the final days of my mother's life.

Over and over, I silently asked myself what would have happened if I hadn't come by. If I hadn't absentmindedly forgotten to drop off my itinerary the day before. No one would have found her for at least another day. I had spoken to all her friends earlier, and they promised to visit and call, but they hadn't that day. Her phone log was empty. I probably wouldn't have called until I was on my way to the airport just to check in and say goodbye.

I searched my memory for what she was wearing the day before since she was fully dressed when I got to her house. Had she been sitting on that toilet all night? The only consolation is that strokes are painless. At least she wasn't suffering for all those unknowable hours.

I'm convinced it was kind of a cosmic or divine intervention. Daddy, Lynnette, and Joanna coaxed me to her house that day. The same way Daddy's spirit coaxed me, Mommy, and my sister's husband, Todd, to the hospital the day my sister went septic. Mysteriously, we all arrived in the middle of a weekday within minutes of each other at a time when none of us would have normally been there. It was as if the energy of those we had loved and lost exerted an unseen force that put us where we needed to be.

Mommy slipped into a deep, deep sleep. As promised, the doctors gave her medicine to lessen the potential for swelling. Judy, Clair, and I stayed until very late and then went our separate ways. Me home to an empty house not knowing whether my mother would live through the night.

The next day, Ralph sat with me at the hospital. He pulled me aside and placed his hands on my shoulders. Looking me in the eyes, he said, "I want you to go on your trip. You should be with your husband. We got this. We'll stay with your mother."

I didn't know what to say. Here she was, lying in a near coma, and he was insisting that I selfishly travel thousands of miles away from where I needed to be.

"Thanks, Ralph, but I can't do that to you. She's my responsibility."

But he wouldn't let it go. He continued to insist that I go. "If something happens, you can get on a plane and come back home. Clairees and I can handle this. You deserve a break. Go be with your husband."

The stroke happened on a Tuesday. Or at least that's when I discovered her. Ralph and I spent all day Wednesday by her side, watching her sleep. She'd wake ever so slightly so that they could draw her blood and fall right back into a deep, deep slumber.

Fred texted me photos that seemed like he and our friends were having a great time, but later, Val, who was there with Fred, told me that he was not.

On Wednesday night, I decided to take Ralph up on his offer. Sometimes, when people make such generous offers, you insult them if you turn them down. Or maybe he would have been relieved if I did.

Mommy was in the safest possible place if anything happened to her. Besides, all I could do was sit and stare at her, watching for signs of improvement.

I'm not a big traveler, and I don't have much experience traveling alone or navigating airline protocol. Traveling abroad by myself was beyond my comfort zone, but I managed to get myself to London on my own.

I met Matt and Marci at Heathrow Airport, and we flew to Edinburgh to connect with Fred, Val, and Josh. We immediately rented cars and drove to Oban. There, we began one of the best vacations I've ever experienced. The scenery. The food. The people we met. We stayed in a little village outside of town in a big house that could accommodate all twelve of us. There was a small tavern on the property called The Barn. It was where we ended most of our nights, drinking with new friends, listening to local music, and joking about the fact that this was the most black folks the people of Oban had ever seen at one time.

I called home every day. I spoke to Clairees or Ralph, whichever one took that day's shift. A few days into the trip, Clairees texted me a photo of Mommy awake and sitting in the chair next to her bed. The brain swelling danger had passed, and she was getting better. What a relief. I wasn't sure until that moment that I wasn't going to get a call that would force me to travel back to the States. That photo gave me the freedom to enjoy the rest of our trip, only needing to make my daily check-in calls.

One afternoon, as Fred and I explored the quaint village, my phone rang. It was Mrs. Carter, a family friend that I had known since I was a small child living in West Philadelphia. She was calling to check on Mommy.

"She's fine, but I'm in Scotland. Ralph and Clairees are watching over her."

"You did go!" she exclaimed.

I was caught completely off-guard by the joy in her voice. I expected to hear disappointment on the other end of the phone. I was prepared for that condemning tone that inferred that I had shirked my responsibilities by leaving Mommy to suffer alone.

"Kyle, I am so happy you went on your trip. I know how much this trip meant to you and Fred. I won't keep you. Have a wonderful time. We'll talk when you get back."

I continued through the sloping streets of this adorable town, processing what had just happened. Mommy had shared so many stories with me about the sacrifices Mr. and Mrs. Carter made to care for their aging ailing parents. How could they be so forgiving about my decision to leave Mommy in the hospital and travel halfway around the world? All this time, I had been carrying the weight of assumptions that turned out to be so wrong.

During the week, we traveled to Skye, one of Scotland's most beautiful and scenic regions. We spent the night and drove back to Oban the next day in a constant downpour. It was the rainiest day of a very rainy trip. It didn't matter. We were on vacation. We were with friends we adored and having a great time.

The drive back to Oban took us through a town called Kyle of Lochalsh. The town's name means "strait of the foaming loch." Kyle can also mean sound, channel, or narrow sea stretch. I had no idea what my name meant until that day. How did an African American family in Philadelphia name their daughter Kyle in 1961? They told me they named me after Kyle Roat, Sr., a football player who played for the Giants. His son, Kyle Roat, Jr., was a well-known soccer player. All my life, I knew they wanted a boy. When I was born, they didn't bother to find a girl's name. They stuck with Kyle.

I read somewhere once that Kyle meant handsome in Gaelic. That's what I'd say when asked. But now, standing some five thousand miles away from where I was given this name, I was in a place that carried the true history of the moniker I hated when I was young. It was too unusual and easy to make fun of. Because of it, people often assume I'm a man. But today, on a trip that I might not have taken, I was surrounded by signs that read, "Kyle of Lochalsh Woolens." "Kyle Pharmacy." "Kyle Art Market." "Kyle Hotel." It was a sign that I was where I was supposed to be. Taking care of Mommy was important, but so was taking care of myself.

I felt the strong connection to my family while in that very place. They saw beyond the boundaries of their own lives and traditional labels and positioned me to live in the world. I don't think they were conscious of this, but by virtue of the name they chose, I was forced to live out an unusual life, not bound by anyone's expectations except theirs. I silently hoped in that moment that I made them proud. I hoped my father's spirit was watching, proudly seeing how far his vision stretched me.

We finished our trip off with a quick eighteen-hour stay in Edinburgh and then flew home and back to reality. Back to figure out what was next on the path stroke was laying out before me.

CHAPTER 23

We returned from Scotland on a Sunday. The next day, I visited Mommy, who was still in the hospital in Trenton. They told me she'd be released the next day. It had been nearly two weeks since the latest stroke. She was alert, but aphasia had her firmly in its grip. The only words she could say were "no," "eminy," and "anferny." She had lost everything she fought to regain on her right side. Her right arm, leg, and face didn't respond to her commands. She would once again require extensive rehabilitation.

The next day, they loaded her into a medical transport vehicle and drove her back down the highway and back to acute rehab in Marlton. I had hoped I'd seen the last of this facility, but what I hoped for didn't matter.

I trusted that they could work their magic again. We came back from the last stroke. We'll come back from this one. That's what I truly believed. The brain has vast regions of unused real estate. Paths could be reestablished in undamaged parts of her brain. Or had too much damage been done? How much can one person's brain handle?

I loaded up the dorm-style closet with the only clothes she wore anymore. This time, there wasn't the deluge of cards, flowers, and stuffed animals. The vast majority of her friends had moved on and, as is to be expected, didn't see the urgency in visiting and rallying behind her. Mommy's incapacities had become everyday stuff, and attention to it was considered optional.

Some of her friends did stick by her through this setback. Ralph, Violet, and Albertha were the most dedicated. They continued to visit. They called to check on me. They even brought her treats. But most people had fallen away. They had returned to their own priorities.

I returned to my routine of visiting daily, but I'd come later in the day and leave at the end of visiting hours.

I posted a few times on CaringBridge. But one post earned me a nasty rebuke from one of Mommy's longtime friends. I had shared that unlike the previously lengthy rehab stay, I might not be at the hospital when they visited. Mommy's friend decided to remind me of all the things my mother had done for me. She let me know, in no uncertain terms, that I should be ashamed of myself for letting up on the gas, even if only a little.

I tried to shake that comment off, but I couldn't. It was one comment from one person out of so many others who praised me for how well I looked after Mommy. Why do we only let the bad stuff stick? We brush off the compliments as if we don't deserve them, but harsh, ugly criticism rattles around in our brain, spewing doubt all over our good judgment.

Maybe I shouldn't have made my plans public. After all, it's no one else's business how I choose to spend my caregiving time. It had been eighteen months since my life had been hijacked. I had sacrificed so much, making Mommy a priority every day.

I told myself I was coming to terms with Mommy's right to choose. She chose to stop taking her medications. She chose not to continue to do the work that would have increased her ability to function independently. She was a big girl who made decisions that landed her where she was. I was getting out of the way of her wrecking ball of stubbornness. I needed to think about my self-preservation, even if it was met with scorn.

This stroke was different. Previously, Mommy made a little progress every day. Some days when I arrived, I'd find her alert, eating dinner and watching TV. Other days, I'd find her in a dead sleep, not even waking to greet me. Coming to just barely for the nurses and aides who were tending to her.

During my conferences with her care team, they said there were days Mommy just couldn't get out of bed. They said it was her brain healing from the extreme trauma of the last stroke. There were also many days that she just wasn't capable of going to therapy.

Then she stopped making noticeable progress. I knew that once they marked that on her chart, her rehab days were numbered.

Her speech never returned. Any time I'd meet someone new on her care team, they'd ask, "Are you Emily?"

"There is no Emily," I'd reply. "She has aphasia, and that's all she can say."

I was surprised by how few people in such a facility understood that. Wasn't it on her chart? Didn't they read it thoroughly to understand what they were dealing with? Apparently not.

The rehab staff were as patient and kind as they were the first two times she was there. They dealt with acute cases every day, and they seemed less bolted to their assumptions about how someone should act. They knew how unpredictable stroke could be. They also knew that there were many ways that it manifested. They didn't lose their temper or punish her for what on the surface seemed like laziness.

When it was time for her to step down to subacute care, we returned to the same facility in Moorestown. I felt I had done my homework before, and she had a very good experience there. But this time, things had changed.

They wheeled her into a very spacious room at the end of the corridor. At first, I thought this was great. More room for visitors. But it quickly became clear that this was not special in a good way. Her roommate was psychotic. She was white, in her fifties it would appear, and alone. No one came to visit during the two weeks we shared the space with her. She required an attendant twenty-four hours a day. She would scream, get violent, and wander over to Mommy's side of the room often. Sometimes when I arrived, she was sitting with her attendant in the common area just outside the room, but when dinner time came, she and her erratic behavior returned.

Every day, there was a different attendant. Some could control her better than others. But when she behaved for a good stretch, their focus turned to the TV or their cell phone and not paying attention to whatever trouble she was getting into. Sometimes, when the roommate would try take Mommy's food or a piece of her clothing,

I'd have to search the floor for her attendant who wandered away or refocus their attention on the task for which they were being paid.

On the days that Mommy was alert, she'd look at me and roll her eyes when her roomie acted up. Mommy had always been a very tolerant person. She could forgive and tolerate the behavior and habits of just about anyone, unless you were one of her immediates, of course. Even though Mommy didn't show any evidence that she felt threatened, I knew this couldn't be a good environment for her, so I requested she be moved to another room.

Mommy continued to get extremely drowsy some days, resisting the aides who came to dress her in the morning. That meant she missed therapy. I believed that the doctors were right when they said it was her brain's way of directing energy to its healing. But on those days, the aides didn't bother to get her up to go the bathroom or check to see if she had gone in the bed.

The staff also wasn't making any special effort to make sure she ate. That's the kind of thing they mark in a chart, or at least they did at some of the facilities she'd been in. If someone doesn't eat, that's a sign that something may be wrong. She clearly wasn't getting the nutrition she needed. If I asked, she would tell me she didn't like the food. So I'd bring food from home, but she wouldn't touch that either.

Finally, a few days after my request, they moved Mommy to another room down the hall. It was a smaller shared room with an elderly lady who had apparently gotten on the staff's last nerve. They mostly ignored her calls and came only when they were obligated.

"My son is a doctor," she told me with great pride in her voice. "If he knew how they were treating me here, he'd have this place shut down."

I met her son one day when he came in to discuss his mother's complaints. Nothing changed after that.

On weekends, I'd plan something special. For instance, she loved the Madagascar movies—so much so that she made "I Like to Move It Move It," the ringtone on the old flip phone. So I bought *Madagascar 3: Europe's Most Wanted*, and we watched it together on my laptop with popcorn to add a dose of specialness to the experience.

One of the hardest days came when on a Saturday afternoon, I arrived around two-thirty and found Mommy lying in a pool of urine. I immediately went looking for the nurse aide assigned to Mommy's room.

"My shift is about to end," she quickly blurted out when I asked her to clean Mommy up, change the sheets, and put fresh clothes on her. But she wasted no time informing me that she was not interested in taking on a new project before she clocked out.

I never understood or had the luxury to think about my work this way. My entire life, I was a salaried employee, which meant the words "clocking out" carried no meaning. But hourly workers are cut from a different cloth and often punished if they work overtime without permission.

"Your mother didn't want to get up. When they tell us that, we don't force them," she explained very matter-of-factly. There was no remorse. She offered no apology. She spoke with swarthy conviction and no fear of retribution.

"Please get me clean towels, sheets, and your supervisor," I demanded. I was mortified that a young African American girl could be so cavalier about her job. Didn't she know that the system required very little to label her worthless and quickly dispose of her?

I woke Mommy up, helped her out of bed, and wheeled her into the bathroom. I stripped off the soaking wet clothes and washed her from head to toe. She didn't complain. She didn't throw a tantrum and insist on staying in bed. If she was going to do that with anyone, it would have been with me. She willingly complied, even though she was visibly tired.

While I was in the bathroom doing part of the aide's job, she changed the sheets, throwing in lots of attitude along the way. When three o'clock came, she was gone. The supervising nurse came into chat, but she didn't instill me with the confidence that things would change.

"If you continue to have problems, let me know, but…" and out came the excuses. "We're short-staffed on weekends. Sometimes things fall through the cracks, and I'm very sorry. I'll keep an eye out in the future."

When I spoke to the supervisor, I asked the horrible questions that rushed through my head. "How long had she been lying there for the urine to actually pool up? It has saturated the adult diaper and her underwear and had leaked all the way through to the mattress. Did no one check her throughout the day to see this developing? Everybody goes to the bathroom. It's not like this would have been unexpected. When someone says they don't feel like getting up, isn't in the staff's responsibility to at least make sure they're clean and safe?"

I got no satisfactory answers. I hoped that the conversation alone would have some impact on the future. But sadly, I was mistaken. It happened frequently, on all those days when Mommy's healing brain drained her energy and the staff just complied as if she was capable of the calling the shots.

Soon after, I began getting complaints from the physical therapy staff. "Your mother won't do the exercises. She refuses to try anything. She just says no."

I was called in to discuss this with the social worker who asked me to come in during the day to watch Mommy in class and to help encourage her.

"Does it hurt when you try to do what they ask?" I tried to get the answers they couldn't.

"No," she replied.

"Are you tired?"

"No."

"Do you understand that this is the only way you'll get better? You were great at this before, and you saw how much it helped."

"Eminy," she'd say, looking at me out of the side of her eye with a willful stare that spoke volumes. A stare that shouted "Leave me alone." For some reason, she was done with them, and I couldn't figure out why.

The strangeness continued. Mommy began laughing at the most inappropriate things. Her laugh was loud and piercing. She'd laugh when someone screamed out in pain. When the nurse came in to draw blood. When someone stumbled or dropped something.

Mommy laughed particularly hard when I suffered a hot flash. Whenever I began peeling off clothes and furiously fanning myself, she'd look at me and break out into a loud sustained laughter. Being amused by my suffering wasn't really new. The difference was that her piercing wail was disrupting the quiet skilled nursing unit, and people reacted.

One of the doctors pulled me aside and said, "We don't know what's wrong with your mother. She's been laughing inappropriately, and it's a problem." She spoke to me as if I had the answers.

"Is this something you've seen before?" The doctor looked puzzled and dismayed. It was like they were looking for an answer that would let them off the hook. As if I'd confirm that Mommy was a bad seed and their anger at her was justified.

I went home that night and consulted Dr. Google. I searched "Strokes and inappropriate laughter," and several listings came up immediately. Inappropriate reactions are known to be associated with stroke. Shouldn't a doctor in a rehab facility know this?

And the hits just kept on coming. They complained that Mommy didn't want to go to bed at 8:00 p.m. It appears to be standard practice in nursing facilities to start getting residents ready for bed right after dinner. On our first stay, Mommy wanted me to put her to bed, and visiting hours were over at eight. So she was in step with what staff expected. But she'd lie in bed for the rest of the night watching TV. She may have been in bed, but she wasn't asleep.

This time, she didn't want to get ready for bed at eight o'clock. She wanted to stay dressed in her wheelchair until she was tired and ready to go to sleep. Apparently, this defiant behavior was too much for them to handle. They'd report to me that she didn't want to go to bed until eleven. To which I'd respond, "She's a grown woman and can determine when she wants to go to bed. I really don't see what the big deal is."

Another example of odd behavior was her insistence that she sleep in only her bra and panties. She even refused to wear her silky caftans. She seemed unnerved by the fact that the door to her room was always open, and anyone who walked by could see her in her underwear. One wrong move and out came the lady parts. This was a tremendous departure from the person my mother was before the stroke. She'd never let strangers see her in her underwear; that is, unless she was trying on clothes in one of Loehmann's notoriously wide-open fitting rooms.

On the days Mommy was awake enough to go to therapy, she still dug in her heels. And the staff became more and more frustrated, as did I. Medicare was paying a tidy sum for her to be there, and they were the experts. I sure wasn't. Was I wrong to believe that they should have had other tricks up their sleeve to get her to cooperate? I felt more like they just didn't care and that the whole place was built on a culture of not caring. I could sense a lack of empathy and compassion everywhere.

I chose this place because Mommy had such a wonderful experience the first time. Now even the building itself was quickly losing its charm. It had been less than a year, and the French provincial décor was visibly duller. The rooms showed so much wear and tear. Mommy complained constantly about the food. And unfortunately, winter was approaching, so I couldn't even take her outside to see the horses. The lovely Equestrian Overlook, the seating area with large windows with a view of the horse farm, had become a storage area cluttered with beds, equipment, and other things while they worked on renovations. The gild was off the lily. From top to bottom, inside and out, the place that we had once found comforting was gone.

Since Mommy wasn't making progress, I had to figure out where she'd go once they were done with her. Could I really ask Fred to take her in again? There was no end in sight to her staying with us if she moved back in. She wasn't ever going to get healthy enough to go back to her own house. She would just plant herself in our family room, never ever making any effort to get back what she lost. This was not the fate to which I wanted to surrender.

I asked the social worker if Mommy was a candidate for assisted living. At that point, it was easier to hold on to my faith in their ability to take care of her than to be rushed into making a decision about what would come next. I figured a temporary move to assisted living would buy me some time to figure out a longer-term plan. But I had unwittingly opened a door to the possibility of paying for

Mommy to stay there. Their focus on getting her better changed almost immediately to getting her money.

The social worker called in the marketing director to give me a tour. He said they thought she would do fine in their assisted living unit. But I was still feeling a good deal of angst about how they had already treated her, so I didn't commit to anything. I also couldn't shake the feeling that I was being shystered.

A few days later, my friend Sylvia, who worked for Bayada, called. "Did you know they're discharging your mother on Thanksgiving Day?"

It was the week before Thanksgiving, and no, I didn't know. Angrily, I asked, "How on earth could anyone think it was a good idea to discharge someone on Thanksgiving Day? That's just ridiculous!"

I felt like we were being punished for something.

The next care conference was charged with negative energy. Sitting in a small conference room, they laid out their argument to the two of us.

"We really don't think your mother is taking her therapy seriously. Plus, she's become difficult, and she refuses to comply with the therapists."

"Okay," I said as Mommy gave them her best mean stare. "What is she doing?"

"She's just not trying, and some days, she refuses to get out of bed. We can't help her if she doesn't want the help. The therapists don't think there's anything else they can do for her."

I had been called to the principal's office to hear how horrible my bully child was behaving. I didn't know who to believe, them or my mother, who sat giving them looks that seem to imply they were lying. This was far from what I expected from a facility to which I was now considering paying cash to continue her care. We were now about to become the customer, not Medicare. I expected that to mean something.

Their arrogance seemed fueled by the assumption that we had no other options. It was as if they assumed we would blindly follow their recommendations because they were the best game in town, and we wouldn't bother to go anywhere else. They read me as desperate not to take Mommy home.

They read me wrong.

CHAPTER 24

The therapy team was done with Mommy. The sales team was mentally banking our dollars. I instantly reacted to what I felt was coercion. They stood to benefit in cold, hard cash if Mommy moved into assisted living. No more negotiating and reporting to Medicare. I'd be writing the check every month, no questions asked. They took my patience with their vapid care to mean that I was still willing to give them another chance. They gambled, and they lost.

I immediately called Fred and asked who I needed to speak to about transferring Mommy to a different facility right around the corner. I had taken a tour of it after Mommy's first stroke, but at the time, their skilled nursing department was housed in a dank, dingy basement. Even though they were the top-rated senior living community, I couldn't see putting Mommy there.

But they had since built a new unit that rivaled the best five-star hotels. There was a dining room on every floor. A great contrast to the way the other facility singled out temporary patients who had to eat in their rooms. The rooms were spacious, and all the furniture was brand-new. Each cluster of five or six rooms had a cozy common area with a TV and a balcony that overlooked their manicured grounds. It was perfect.

Once I gave their medical director permission to visit Mommy to assess her needs, he went immediately. Shortly after, I got a call telling me they had a room for her. I was thrilled. Not only because she'd be moving into this new, immaculately appointed, highly rated facility, but because I could use her moving up to taunt the marketing team. We weren't as desperate as they thought. We were moving to the competition.

I went to her room that afternoon and packed up all her things. They weren't able to find the social worker during the forty-five minutes it took me to execute Mommy's getaway. I loaded her into my car for the two-minute drive to a new, nicer rehab community. As I waited for someone to help unload her, my phone rang. It was the social worker who I had come to mistrust.

"I'm sorry, Ms. Ruffin, but we were planning to move your mother this week to our assisted living unit," she said, trying to be sweet yet barely hiding her annoyance. "I was really surprised when I heard you had taken her out of here today. Where will she be?"

I shared the name of Mommy's new home with my chest puffed out and a tone that didn't hide my disappointment in their inability to serve us. I imagined her mentally recalculating who she thought we were and how much we could afford.

"Oh." She paused. "That's a nice place, but so is our facility, and we were preparing a room for her."

"That's not my problem," I said to myself, wishing I had the balls to say it out loud.

She responded to my silence with her offer of assistance in the future.

"Thank you and goodbye," I said.

I immediately began writing a letter to their corporate office in North Jersey in my head. I had threatened to write letters in the past when I felt wronged and didn't follow through. But this time, I was determined.

"Mommy, you know this is one of Fred's clients? That means you should love the food." I stayed through dinner. She picked at her meal. I thought she was just tired from the frenzy of activity. I kissed her goodbye and went home to write and send my angry letter. No one bothered to reply.

"No, I'm not Emily. My name is Kyle. There is no Emily. That's all she can say." That's how I now introduced myself to the staff and new roommates she'd have throughout her stay.

The medical team was able to get Mommy's therapy extended, even though according to the facility we fled, her benefits had been exhausted. On therapy days, they'd take Mommy into the common area outside her room and run through some exercises. Rather than roll her back into her room, they kept her out there so she wouldn't just sit alone staring at her TV for the rest of the day. Instead, she got to interact with other residents and staff. She watched others in therapy and engaged with staff who sometimes took their lunch breaks in that same area.

Her innate need to be in the presence of people was being served in a new and important way. She would never have asked to be taken out of her room, but she didn't insist on going back into solitude. Instead, she seemed to become part of the community. They talked to her, and she responded as best she could. And being in the beautiful living room area rather than in the tight confines of her room where there was limited seating made my visits more pleasant.

Unfortunately, we struggled with the food there too. It was becoming painfully clear that she just didn't have her old appetite. Mommy had always loved food. Before the stroke, she enjoyed experimenting with new cuisines and always savored her meals, mindful of every chew and swallow to the point of becoming the butt of jokes. Ralph's late brother, Bill, used to say that after the first session, she'd bail, which meant writhing back and forth in a way that sped up her digestion so she could eat more.

After the second stroke, she had developed oral thrush, a white film that covered her tongue completely. They gave her medicine, which eventually cleared it up, but it seemed to permanently affect her taste buds.

She also started a long stubborn streak of refusing to take her medicine.

At the previous facility, they had inserted a feeding tube to make sure she got the basic nutrition her body needed. I secretly convinced the nurses to use the tube to sneak in medicine. Each night, the nurse would come into the room to flush the feeding tube to keep it clean and clear. Inside the liquid were the dissolved pills Mommy needed to control her arrhythmia, her blood pressure and viscosity, her borderline diabetes, and her seizures.

We fooled her like that for quite some time, but eventually the feeding tube would have to be removed. It's not something that's recommended for the long-term. It had already been in too long, but that would mean we had no way to ensure she was getting the medicine she so badly needed.

I began bringing DVDs from her house so she could watch movies in the common area. The DVD player never seemed to be in use, so we claimed it. She watched her favorites over and over until she got sick of them. The movies became a bit of a social draw. Sometimes residents in the other rooms would come watch with her.

Movies were even a draw for one unexpected guest. I strolled in late one afternoon to find Fred in his suit and tie, sitting with Mommy, watching *The Devil Wears Prada*. He had visited his client and team that day and decided to pay a rare visit to his mother-in-law. It was a strange scene. She in her wheelchair, him in one of the cushioned armchairs from the four-seat table, which he had turned toward the TV. They were immersed in the story on the screen. I could tell he hadn't planned to stay for the whole movie because he still had his coat on. I think he was going to duck in and duck out before I got there, but my husband is a sucker for a poignant human drama. Even ones he's seen several times before.

It was nice to see this brief bonding moment. Fred and Mommy had a good relationship as in-laws go, even though he didn't really help take care of her. He did resent a lot of the same things I resented about her, but he never showed that to her. I always got caught between him and her when she'd make a request that we both thought was ridiculous. If I asked him to do her a favor, he'd launch into a speech about why he wouldn't and then flat-out refuse. Then she'd ask him the very same question, and he would comply. I hated how bad that made me look, so eventually I'd just get her to ask him directly. If I had asked him to come with me to watch a movie with Mommy, the answer would have most certainly been no.

Each day, the staff would fill me in on what Mommy did the night before. They were all extremely pleasant and attentive. Her favorite was Hava. She had a beautiful round Turkish face, long dark flowing hair, and a lovely warm accent. She called Mommy "My Paula."

"What does my Paula need?"

"Did my Paula enjoy her dinner?"

"Last night, my Paula watched Madagascar again."

"My Paula is a night owl. She doesn't like to go to bed when everyone else does."

"That's okay," Hava would say. "I love my Paula. She's fun."

Hava played an important role in bringing joy to Mommy in a very unexpected way. She made Mommy feel special. She'd notice when Mommy got a new outfit. She'd praise her for any progress she made. She'd tell me how great Mommy was in front of her, and that really boosted Mommy's spirits.

Stroke changes people in unimaginable ways. I wish I knew what was at work behind the most fascinating change I witnessed. For her entire life, she had been terrified of birds, no matter how small. When she was a small child visiting family in South Carolina, a mean, persistent chicken chased her, leaving an indelible mark on her psyche. Birds were forever the enemy, so much so that she wouldn't watch the *Wizard of Oz* because of the flying monkeys.

But when Hava introduced her to the parakeet couple in the main living area, Mommy became obsessed. They were colorful and talkative, especially the male. The female loved building nests. She would take slivers of paper that people handed her through the slats in the cage. After carefully tearing them into even smaller strips, she'd take them into their private space, where she busily created a home for her family.

For a good long stretch, every single time I visited, Mommy insisted that I take her to visit the birds. They *were* adorable, but could this be the same person who was terrified by the birds that might fly over her head at Home Depot or Lowes?

When their handler came to clean the cage, Mommy got up close and personal. Some of the staff would even take the male out of the cage and place it close to Mommy. One day, I was treated to the strangest thing of all. Mommy let them put the bird on her head. It walked around on her wig long enough for me to snap a few photos with my phone. She smiled and laughed the entire time. There was no sign of fear, not even a wince when his tiny clawed feet balanced on her head as she tried to look up and smile for the camera.

I showed these pictures to family and friends, and they were astounded. Every single person who knew my mother knew about the intense fear she had carried most of her seventy-one years. Their responses were consistent.

"Who is this woman?"

"That's not the Paula we know."

"She's deathly afraid of birds. This is freaky!"

The therapy staff worked diligently with Mommy, and she was once again able to walk using a device that opened up like a folding chair with a strip along the top onto which she could hold. I video-taped her in action, documenting her great progress to share with friends who called occasionally to ask about her.

It seemed like we were once again moving forward. I began to wonder if we were back on the road to full recovery. Could she really come back from this abyss? Could she recover from a devastating stroke that only months ago felt like the end? Is she stronger than we gave her credit for?

Every week, a lady from a local choir group would make her rounds, visiting people and singing to or with them. She was a petite, older white woman with a falsetto voice that likely carried many important tunes within her choir. She brought her book of hymns and a small round tuning whistle that she used to set the starting note for each song.

The first day I arrived during a singing session, which usually lasted about twenty to thirty minutes, the songstress asked me for names of songs that Mommy might want to sing. Up until that point, she had been guessing since Mommy couldn't name the songs herself. I chose songs I remember hearing as a child in church. "Soldiers of the Cross," "How Great Thou Art," "I Surrender All," and "Just a Closer Walk With Thee." These were the songs that also played on the stereo in our family room every Sunday morning. I knew them well, but Mommy knew them better.

As the woman sang, Mommy joined in. Her words were slurred, but she was clearly singing the right ones. She wasn't just repeating "Eminy." She was singing. "We are climbing Jacob's ladder. We are climbing Jacob's ladder. Soldiers of the cross. Every rung goes higher,

higher. Every rung goes higher, higher. Every rung goes higher, higher. Soldiers of the cross."

I couldn't believe what I was hearing. Mommy was singing actual words. My heart sparked with hope. Maybe this is how we would overcome aphasia this time! One of the therapists who happened to be hanging around that day told me that singing comes from a different part of the brain than speaking. That part of Mommy's brain was not damaged by the stroke. She recommended that we try getting her to sing whatever she was trying to say.

We began with trying to get her to sing "My name is Paula." She sang the words, but it was a struggle. It was as if the songs she'd known since childhood were so firmly etched into her brain that she could access that information with little effort. Just as before, the harder she tried, the less she was able to control what came out of her mouth.

She wanted to talk again. I could see it in her eyes. But her brain was now so damaged that rebuilding the pathways to speech would take so much more work than the last time.

Mommy's physical recovery had slowed, which meant there would be no more Medicare-covered therapy. Sadly, they use metrics to determine whether a person is worth investing in. Once the sand is through their payer's hourglass, the resources go away, and the people move on.

Mommy would receive no more physical or speech therapy, and her stay was no longer covered. If she were to remain, she would have to pay the full rate out of pocket. And since she was at one of the best facilities in the state, the cost of staying on the skilled nursing floor would be hefty.

Part of me understood why this was happening. Resources are limited, and the line needs to be drawn somewhere. But when the sands of the hourglass empty for someone you love and are caring for, it feels personal, no matter how many times you go through it. It always feels like no one cares and that you're all alone in believing that our fellow human beings would want nothing but the best for us. But the reality is that to every person who is part of the vast health care system—the cast of thousands who are not in the room to see

Mommy's face—she was just a number, or more likely the unique combinations of ones and zeros that came together to determine her fate.

Mommy developed a close relationship with an older woman who had moved into the room across the hall. Mary also had trouble speaking.

They looked out for one another, and in spite of their challenges, they were somehow able to communicate. It was as if their maladies gave them access to another dimension that we who can speak don't understand. They were an adorable team. Mary was much older than Mommy, frail, tiny, and spoke so quietly that I had to put my ear inches away from her mouth to hear her. Mommy was tall, imposing, and loud whenever she laughed.

Mary's family brought her an iPad with an app that she could use to type out what she wanted to say. She was slow but accurate, which impressed both me and Mommy, especially since Mary was so clearly not of the tech generation.

Inspired by Mary, I installed a keyboard app on my iPad to see if Mommy could use it to communicate, but she just couldn't get the hang of it. Because of her aphasia, she would type the wrong letters the same way she'd write the wrong letters. We tried over and over, but Mommy was never able to use the alphabetical or the QWERTY keyboard.

She had never gotten around to learning how to type. She intended to. I once found a how-to video beside her bed at home, but it was too late now. It was like me trying to learn how to swim at forty. There comes a time when natural instincts are harder to tap into and new habits become more difficult to form. After a few weeks, I surrendered to Mommy's frustration and stopped pushing her.

Each evening, Mommy and Mary watched movies together. Mary always wanted to see something old in black and white. Those were hard to come by, so I'd cue up one of my favorites, Dr. Zhivago. Although it wasn't black and white, it was old and a wonderfully epic, beautifully filmed classic.

I have watched Dr. Zhivago over and over. I love the story and the memory of Mommy and Daddy going to see it when I was a child in the sixties. They left Lynnette and me with a babysitter as they headed out to the Main Line to the movie theater across from Strawbridge's department store. I don't recall ever talking to them about the movie. I was only five or six when they saw it. But I do remember that there was something very adult about the film, something that made it not for children's eyes. It conjured up feelings and childhood memories that clung to me. Watching Dr. Zhivago made me feel closer to Mommy and Daddy somehow. I was finally in on the movie's dirty little secrets of older men pushing themselves on teenage girls and extramarital affairs. In the nineties, when I finally saw it for the first time, those things seemed so tame. Not only is Dr. Zhivago an incredible movie in and of itself, but our shared experience decades apart drew out the emotions of a coming of age moment for me. That movie holds a magic that will always transport me back into the little girl watching Mommy and Daddy leave for their date night.

Mommy's spirits were good. She was in a good place, and I was happy. But another swell was building, and I needed to get into position to swim parallel to the shoreline.

CHAPTER 25

My attorney, kept me updated on the progress to sell Uncle Charlie's house. I was also painfully aware of their efforts to evict the woman who was squatting in Uncle Abner's house, living in squalor with holes in the roof where rainwater poured in and rotted the wallpaper. The mother had moved out, but the daughter had allowed a perfectly good house to decline into dilapidation. Brad sent me photos. It was inconceivable that someone could live in these conditions, even if the house was free.

The attorneys were also working to determine if Abner and Daisy had ever been adopted. If they were, my uncles and cousins would share what was left over from Abner's estate. In an ironic twist, as my father's only living child, I would have been an heir to the money my mother spent. In Pennsylvania, family inheritance bypasses widowed spouses and goes only to blood or legally recognized children. I was just as much a victim as everyone else I was fighting against, yet loyalty to Mommy trumped any of that. Feeling robbed could not get in my way of being the shield that protected Mommy from any backlash.

I received word from my attorney that Uncle Edgar's lawyer and he had negotiated an agreement. He called to ask if I would agree to sell my mother's house and turn over $154,000 from the sale to reimburse Uncle Abner's estate.

I read through the documents they sent that laid out the details. I understood the words, but not what might lie between the lines. After I had another attorney review the agreement and assure me that everything was sound, I signed and returned it, feeling the full weight of being the last person in my immediate family responsible for handling family business. I alone had just committed to selling the house that sheltered no others except my family since it was built in 1971.

For decades, that house was a place of safety and celebration. It was the crowning achievement of all my parents' accomplishments. The manifestation of Daddy's hard work and passion for living a good life. It was where Pierre, our crazy cocker spaniel, would voraciously bark at company as they tried to leave. It was where both parents threw each other surprise birthday parties. It was where Lynnette and I took our prom pictures and where I got married the first time. The house was a loyal member of the family that was always there anytime we needed it.

I was losing that family member and closing the door on any possibility that Mommy would return to her beloved home to live in relative independence.

Selfishly, I didn't tell Mommy. I thought it would just make her sad, and I didn't want to deal with her emotions. I just wanted to marinate in my own. It was hard enough knowing what I had ahead of me. As much as I wanted her to suffer along with me, given that she created this crisis, I also knew that adding her anguish would have served no one.

Shortly after, the facility's social worker sat me down and suggested I consider admitting Mommy permanently. "You'll be able to enjoy your mother rather than constantly serve her," she said.

I laughed. "I will always be her servant. That's why I'm on this earth. Mommy has made that clear."

I cringed at the idea of making another major life decision for her. What would her friends say? Would they be disappointed in me, wondering why I didn't take her back to my house? Thinking about what others would say created its own paralyzing anxiety. Here I was again at a crossroads. I had to choose between my mother and Fred.

If I took her home, it would be a hardship our marriage was strong enough to survive, but I didn't want to risk it. I also knew how much I needed to keep my life with Mommy and my life with Fred separate. If she came to live with us, I'd *never* get a break. This time, she required way more assistance than before. There would be little to no respite if I had to take full responsibility for her care.

Putting Mommy into a nursing home meant breaking a promise I never made, but one that I never denied in my heart. Before the first stroke, I believed this decision was decades away. I could put it off, and maybe things would change in a way that would mean I didn't have to be the one to choose. In my ideal fantasy, I'd win millions in the lottery and buy a house with guest quarters or an attached mother-in-law suite where she and permanent live-in help would stay. I could spend time with her, keeping her close enough to make us both comfortable but far enough to keep her out of Fred's and my sacred space.

The time for wishful thinking was over. I couldn't put it off any longer. I had to find a permanent place for Mommy to live. She was happy in her lush surroundings, but with great luxury comes a great price tag. Her resources could keep her in this gilded cage for about a year. After that, I would have to find a place that accepted Medicaid while she still had enough in her bank account for a few months of private pay.

When I told her what I was contemplating, she didn't seem upset at all. She just looked at me without any expression. Maybe this decision took some pressure off her too. Since she couldn't hold a conversation, she couldn't tell me if she eventually wanted to go back home. And I don't remember asking.

I stopped consulting her on her major life decisions. I just acted on her behalf, and she just let me. She completely surrendered the hard stuff to me a long time ago. She didn't ask about her house, her car, or her bank account. And I did what I thought was best without any concern for what she might want.

The only time Mommy did express interest in her things was when I'd say I was going to sell her car. She cherished that Mercedes ML320. It was midnight blue with grayish blue seats. It had all the bells and whistles a car could have in 2002. She loved it so much that for the first time since moving into our family house in 1971, she cleared away all the things stored in one side of the garage so she could keep her baby pristine. She even had garage door openers installed. She only drove it on the weekends until the 1999 Mitsubishi Galant she took over after my sister died finally stopped running. When she bought the Mercedes, she said that was the last car she was ever going to buy, and I knew by the way she treated it that she meant it.

Anytime I mentioned selling her baby, she'd become agitated, repeating, "No, no, no, no, no, no, no," shaking her head from side to side, each head swing punctuated with a rhythmic no. So I stopped talking about it.

I took her non-response about now living in a facility to mean she was okay with it. But I was prepared for a fight, like the one I always got when I mentioned the car. I expected her to react in a way that would make it clear that I was to take her in and that would be that. I expected her to exert her parental authority the way she always had and that I would cower and give in. But none of that happened. I was puzzled but relieved.

I began visiting nearby senior living facilities that were convenient for me since I knew I'd be going there often. As her only family, I couldn't bear to know that she might languish for days not seeing me or her friends, whose visits were down to a couple a week.

I settled on the Masonic Home in Burlington. The rooms were large, and she would have her own with no roommate. I liked that. We could even bring furniture from home so that she could be surrounded by things she used to love. It was a little farther away from my house than I would have liked, but in my heart, I knew this was a place she could thrive.

I hatched a plan to keep her in her five-star digs until she had about four to six months of money in her bank account to pay for her care and housing. That amount of money would pave the way for easy admittance to the Masonic Home. By my account, she could live in the lap of luxury until the end of 2013.

But then we got a call that would extend that time. The medical staff recommended that we move Mommy from skilled nursing to assisted living. That came with a thirty percent drop in the monthly fee. She could stay longer and still have enough to go to the Masonic Home with a nice private pay cushion.

Mommy moved upstairs and shared a room with various people from independent living who needed special care from time to time. Even though she couldn't speak, she made fast friends with all of them.

In one of the sweetest ironic twists, Hava's sister was assigned to Mommy's room. Her name was Emine.

"So you're Emine," I said, gasping and laughing at the same time. "Paula has been looking for you for months!"

Emine was just as sweet and attentive as Hava. They were like angels sent directly from heaven. Their jobs are extremely tough, even backbreaking at times, but both showed nothing but love for the work and the people they cared for.

Meanwhile, the clock was ticking on selling Mommy's house. The documents I signed put a September deadline on completing the sale and reimbursing the estate. It was only February, but on top of all I had to do for her, I was tending to my growing list of clients and staying active with the organizations for which I volunteered. Now I had to clear out forty-two years of cherished memories and carefully sift through the mountains of stuff my mother had neatly hoarded away in every closet, drawer, and open space.

The emotions this new project stirred up were unavoidable. I was angry and sad that all this fell to me, but I was also relieved to clear away another obstacle that stood between me and freedom from worrying about another relic of Mommy's old life. I could rid us of this albatross on my terms without having to deal with resistance brought on by her sentimentality for our family home. Not that I wasn't sentimental, but there was nothing left of our old life there. The people were gone. Now the house stood solely as a monument to things.

CHAPTER 26

After Daddy died in 1995, I tried to convince Mommy to move into a smaller, more manageable house. Instead, she continued to fill this house with souvenirs from her trips abroad and lots and lots of clothes and accessories. It took years, but she finally gave away all of Daddy's clothes. Going through someone's closet means the difficult experience of revisiting a life once lived and lost. Remembering where he last wore that suit. Or that day they were shopping when he bought those shoes. Or the party they were at when he dripped chicken grease on that tie. I understood her delay, but I also wanted her to move on. It was only when she and Ralph began dating four years after Daddy died that she finally found the courage to remove Daddy's things from the house they shared for twenty-four years.

Over the next decade, Mommy filled in all the empty space that getting rid of Daddy's belongings opened up. Shortly after Lynnette died in 2002, Mommy marched over to her apartment and began packing up clothes, jewelry, and photo albums. She called me and insisted that I join her, but I refused. How could I expand my wardrobe with clothes left behind by someone who had suffered the way Lynnette had? The sting of her death was still fresh, and I could see little else than selfish greed in an act my mother insisted was altruistic.

"It will help Todd," Mommy said with a stern rebuke. But I stood my ground.

Todd, my sister's widowed husband, was moving out of the apartment they shared and into a house he had hoped to live a long and happy life with his now-deceased wife. They had begun house shopping just before she died. The apartment he was still in was

Lynnette's long before they met, but they had filled it with material goods that represented their life together.

Mommy didn't see taking Lynnette's things as benefitting from her death. She saw it as lightening Todd's load. That was one of the many ways we saw the world differently. It wasn't as if I felt Mommy preferred things over people. I knew better. If she could have her daughter back, she'd take that over the things she was now gathering up. But my emotions were still at the boiling point after the last days of Lynnette's life became turbulent and pit us against one another.

Leading up to her death, I spent hours on the phone calling around for second opinions and hoping against hope that there was still a way to save my only sister. I finally got her to agree to see another doctor. Mommy and I sat with Lynnette as the doctor callously explained that all that could be done had been and that she was a lost cause. All I could see was this doctor's unwillingness to help my sister because she did this to herself.

"You smoke?" she asked.

"Yes," Lynnette quietly answered.

The doctor's tone was that of someone who believed that since she was a smoker, she got what she deserved. Her disgust was punctuated with an eastern European accent that made her sound dismissive and bothered that we took up her time.

"All I would have done is what the doctors have already done for you," she said while looking at Lynnette's chart and X-rays.

That was the day the light went out in my sister's eyes.

"She said there's nothing else they can do for me," she told her husband, holding back tears as we sat trying to have lunch in a nearby restaurant. As I listened to her, it was clear that she had lost all hope and was consumed with the knowledge that she was going to die. She had been afraid of dying since she was a child. I had known this since the day I found her sitting on the steps in our West Philly home crying her eyes out.

"What's wrong?"

"I'm going to die someday," she blurted out as she cried uncontrollably.

And now I felt responsible for the moment she learned that her life was nearing its end. I felt horribly responsible for exposing my physically and emotionally frail sister to the pain of her fear becoming reality.

I didn't think things could get worse, but they did. A few weeks later at Hazel's son's wedding, Lynnette began exhibiting symptoms of a stroke. Her smile and her gate were noticeably lopsided. The size four suit she had borrowed from me was falling to one side. I insisted on following her home that night. When I described Lynnette's condition to Fred, he made me call her right away. "Can Todd take you to the hospital tonight?" I asked.

"He has to work," she responded. "I feel fine."

"You might feel fine, but something is definitely wrong, Lynnette."

First thing the next morning, Fred and I took her to the hospital, where after sitting in the waiting room for six or seven hours, they revealed that the cancer had spread to her brain. Mommy joined us later after she closed her store. So did my cousin Tony, Clairees, and Doreen's brother, who happened to be in town from Boston.

Radiation treatments quickly followed on top of her chemo. The cancer in her brain was treated successfully, but her immune system was so far gone that her body had nothing with which to fight back. She stopped eating. She refused all the experimental trials the doctors recommended. I begged her to change her mind, but she dug her heels in.

She made it clear that she didn't want any visitors. Even her best friends were asked to stay away. Through the grapevine, girlfriends and relatives with whom she had shared the most intimate parts of her life and who meant the most to her were discouraged from coming to see her. She was tired and frail. Her head was bald and burned from radiation treatments. Lynnette just wanted to be left alone. But that's not how Mommy felt one's last days should be spent.

When the doctors began preparing us for Lynnette's death, against my sister's wishes, Mommy called everyone she knew and asked them to come say goodbye. One afternoon, as I was leaving Lynnette's room, the ex-husband of one of her girlfriends walked in.

"Your mother called me and told me that I should come say goodbye." He was such a random person to visit that I knew Mommy was at home leafing through her phone book for names and numbers of people to share the sad news that the end was near.

For four days in a row, the doctors called saying each time that this was going to be her final day with us. The very last call came on a Monday. I left work immediately and headed straight to the hospital. I walked in to a scene that I knew Lynnette didn't want. Her room was overcrowded with our family and Todd's. My cousin Doreen flew in from Atlanta. Clairees drove up from Maryland, which is where she was living at the time. Todd's large family, brothers, sisters, his mother, all competed for space in Lynnette's hospital room.

When I walked out into the hallway, Mommy was standing with my cousins, mounting a plan to move Lynnette to a different hospital. Not only was she ignoring Lynnette's dying wishes, but she had waited until it was absolutely too late to get serious about helping her daughter.

Feeling overwhelmed and angry, I left not knowing where I was going, but I knew I needed space. One of Todd's brothers followed me, but the closer he got, the faster I walked. I wasn't ready to be consoled. I just wanted to scream and punch things. Mommy had robbed Lynnette of a peaceful end with complete certainty that she was right.

I walked, crying uncontrollably. I walked and walked until I found a hiding spot in the hospital parking garage. I needed to be alone with my anger and disappointment. I needed to be away from the person who hijacked Lynnette's final hours. Mommy found me anyway. When she did, I walked to my car hoping she wouldn't follow, but she stayed on my heels. She got in and tried to explain herself as I continued to sob.

"You're ignoring your own daughter's last wishes!" I screamed. "You knew she didn't want this to become a circus, and you called everyone anyway. Now they're sitting in that room watching Lynnette die. How selfish *are* you?"

"I called everyone because they'd want to say goodbye," she explained calmly.

"What they want doesn't matter! All that matters is what Lynnette wants. Please leave me alone. I need to be alone. Please just go! Please go. Please, please, please go. I can't look at you right now. Just go!" I had never spoken to my mother that way, but I couldn't hold back the avalanche of emotions that were flowing out of me.

Mommy slowly climbed out of the car, leaving me alone to cry it out. I was overwhelmed with the thoughts of losing my sister and the frightening realization that I was being left here with a selfish mother who was now completely my responsibility. I was the only reasonable person left in my family, and I knew on that day that all the important things, all the hard things, would fall on me.

Mommy didn't know how to judge a situation for what it was. Her automatic pilot was guided by family habits and traditions, not by what each unique moment required. I knew in that moment that whatever the future held, I'd never ever be able to count on her to observe the facts and make decisions based in reality. She was a "This is what we've always done" person, and she had no interest in or intention of changing.

Mommy found it easier to rely on tradition. It meant she didn't have to weigh the many options that were actually available to her. She didn't have to look beyond her assumptions. She didn't have to educate herself beyond what she saw on TV or what her friends and family imparted to her. She didn't have to make tough decisions that might turn out to be wrong in the end. She could comfortably say "Well, that was meant to be." The famous last words of someone who is unaware of the power they have to change things.

"I'll leave it in God's hands. Or I'm just going to pray on it." When I hear those phrases, I don't find comfort. I hear the sound of giving up. I hear that I'm not going to test the boundaries of what's possible, even a little bit. I hear "I'm going to ignore my responsibility and ability to play an active role in my own fate."

I could have done that with Mommy's care. I could have left it up to God for her to get better. I could have prayed for a better outcome after the first stroke. I could have succumbed to being a victim dragged down by the sins of my mother. No one would have challenged me, knowing the path I had walked for the last two years, at least not to my face.

Plenty of times, I did pray. Like King Solomon, I prayed for strength and wisdom. God or the powers of the universe answered my prayers by helping me get through some of the toughest days I've ever experienced.

The way I see it, if you're going to leave it in God's hands, he's already looking out for you. He gave us doctors, nurses, lawyers, therapist, educators, researchers, and now the Internet. He is doing his job every day, finding new ways to help us thrive. It's up to us to use what he lays before us to make our own lives better wherever and whenever we can. I needed to believe that. It gave me strength and the perspective I needed to force myself to do the impossible. It powered my ability to take baby steps toward a bigger goal.

This was my self-righteousness, not based on God's direct touch but on using what God gave me and all of us. This is what gave me the energy and the drive to keep pushing through the mud pit of stroke caregiving. If I gave up, the bad stuff would catch up to me, and I'd suffer more. The bad stuff is always there. It never stops chasing you. But when you don't turn around, look it in the eye, and see it for what it is, fear of the unknown, fear of failure, or even fear of success will magnify the bad stuff.

CHAPTER 27

When it came to emptying Mommy's house, I took many, many baby steps. It didn't look like a hoarder lived there, until you looked into every closet and saw that no space had been spared.

In my family, we saved things, even if we tucked them away in the basement and forgot we had them. We might need to use them again, or we might meet someone who could use this perfectly good logoed coffee mug or outfit that no longer fits. I understood the connection Mommy had to these things. Memories came alive with everything I touched. That trip, that funeral, that wedding, that family reunion, that conversation, that holiday, that call in the middle of the night.

It was starting to make sense why she kept shoes that were out of date, trinkets that, to anyone else, meant nothing, foreign money from places she visited, or the cheap figurines from the flea market business she and Daddy ran together for years.

Buried in that need to hold on is the assumption of an endless future. The belief that your life could still go in so many directions and you need to be prepared for every possibility. When you get that call, you'll be happy you saved that flowered notepad, bank pen, and pukka shell necklace. There might come a time when there are no more pens being made, all others are out of ink, and you have the only good one left that can save your life MacGuyver-style. Phew! When that happens, Mommy and Joanna, the mother she inherited this tendency from, would say, "See, I told you not to throw that away!"

Closets in all four bedrooms were filled with clothes. Her bedroom and my sister's walk-in closets housed stacks of shoes in clear plastic boxes so she could easily search for the pair she wanted to wear. This was one of the few organization projects she saw through to the end. At the top of her bedroom closest were stacks and stacks of purses—some old, some new, many from her trips around the world.

The dresser drawer that she had moved into my old room was packed with night clothes, underwear, and jewelry. And of course, there was the bedroom version of the everything drawer. It was the final resting place for trinkets and baubles. The further back they were stuffed into the drawer, the older they were.

She had moved the matching armoire that once served as Daddy's dresser into the office. The doors had been removed, and it was spilling over with random things like a martini-shaped glass filled with mysterious old keys and foreign coins.

The basement had become a graveyard for furniture that once had a starring role somewhere in the house. The old family room sofa and wall unit along with furniture that once spent its summers on the backyard deck. The pool table my parents bought in 1968. The ping-pong table that was a later addition. The surfaces were now covered with leftover merchandise from the years our family sold gift items at area flea markets or clothes that had been left to dry on the clothesline overhead. They were clean but rough-dry, removed from the line to make room for the last load of freshly washed clothes before Mommy's first stroke.

She stored her extensive collection of Christmas ornaments and bulk canned goods in the basement too. The rest of the contents ranged from things she couldn't bring herself to throw out, like old, broken home décor items or raw material from craft projects to things she'd need in the case of nuclear holocaust. Unfortunately, it was all damaged and reeked of mildew because the basement suffered a rare flood just after her first stroke.

Up until the first stroke, she had been trying to maintain this house, rebuking every suggestion I made to move. But everything that was in motion on March 5, 2010, was in suspended animation. Forty-plus-year-old houses deteriorate quickly without lots of tender, loving care.

The crumbling palace that was my parents' pride and joy had become my problem. The roof hadn't been replaced in thirty years. There was evidence that it had been leaking for quite some time. Brown streaks and patches of mold streamed down some of the walls. The worst damage was in the foyer closets, where rank smelling coats were still hanging.

Mommy had replaced the windows throughout the house, but the wood around them was rotting, spilling brown crumbs onto the windowsills through the cracks above. The entire house smelled of water damage and mold, and anyone who visited left smelling the same way.

I called on my friend and real estate agent Alice. She and her daughter and business partner Andrea walked through the house to get a sense for how much we might list it for.

I had done a little online research to see what houses like Mommy's in the same neighborhood were selling for. The work that any family would have to do to move into Mommy's house was already done in the houses that were showing up on Zillow and other real estate websites. I held out hope that a house with such great bones could still fetch a tidy sum, like in the $250,000 range since the renovated homes were selling in the low $300,000s. That would give Mommy a nice cushion once her debt to Abner's estate was paid.

Alice and Andrea went room by room, preparing to give me a number based on how much it would cost for repairs as I nervously stood by. It was like watching Olympic judges calculate deductions for errors in an otherwise perfect gymnastics routine. "The kitchen update will cost x. The mold removal will cost about y. And the house is very close to the highway, which is another deduction. But it's got the original hardwood floors. And that master bathroom is stunning." They guessed the house would sell for about $160,000. I felt that kick squarely in the gut. This was only $5,000 more than what Mommy owed to Abner's estate. And of course, that was before their commission and the termite inspection to determine how bad that damage was.

My childhood house had become a money pit. It had lost tremendous value. It didn't matter though. I would have one less thing to worry about. Instead of dwelling on the bad news, I had to remember the big picture. The important truth was this would mean one less expense to cover. No more money spent on insurance, utilities, and taxes for a house no one was living in. Selling the house eliminated the biggest drain on Mommy's bank account, which was only being fed by her meager social security check.

It was now time to get down to the serious business of clearing out everything that would reveal those beautiful bones. So I mapped out my plan.

Every Monday, I'd spend the entire day working on the house. Clair met me there each week, and we powered through the very daunting process. At first, we'd bounce around from room to room, gathering bags of clothes and shoes, shuffling papers, making emotionally exhausting decisions about what to do with every single thing we touched. Each item required a judgment call. Do I keep it, sell it, give it away, or throw it away?

It felt like we were standing still, making no progress and feeling overwhelmed by the vastness of what still needed to be done. I began to feel the full weight of being left behind by my entire family to determine what would happen to the things they cherished, things that they held onto because of the special way it made them feel.

"You're not throwing away the person. You're throwing away the thing." I had to repeat that to myself over and over. I had to strip myself of the attachment I had to things because they belonged to my family, who were nearly all gone now. I couldn't take it all home. My house was already full of the precious things Fred and I collected. Even if I felt compelled to just pack it up and move it into my house, my type-A husband wouldn't let me past the front door.

I was the judge and the jury for everything Mommy had saved to remind her of the life she had with Lynnette, Daddy, Joanna, Joanna's brother, Uncle Jimmy, her grandparents, Uncle Jim and Aunt Gene (Clair's parents), her best friend, Hazel, even Uncle Charlie. To remind her of the lavish trips she had taken to bucket list places and numerous events celebrating with the family and friends she held dear. The gifts that she couldn't throw away even though she'd never use them.

I thought about that day in the future when someone is going to do this with my things. Fred's nephews and niece are going to throw away that photo of my first cat, Darby, because they won't know how important it was to me. All the furniture that Fred and I spent so much energy and emotion choosing is going to end up in some stranger's college dorm room after being purchased for twenty dollars at a yard sale. Or that Stearns & Foster mattress that we splurged on and slept on for years will end up in a municipal dump covered in bird poop, crawling with maggots or incinerated into ashes. I was overwhelmed with having to make those choices with my family's material things. But as each torturous cleanout day dragged on, cherished belongings lost more and more of their meaning and their value, and I deeply questioned why we bother accumulating so much when it all ends up in the trash.

I returned home one evening complaining that I didn't see how I was going to get this entire house cleaned out. Fred, who had already gone through this with his childhood home, gave me some very good advice.

"Clean one room at a time. When that room is done, move to the next one." He knew how scattered I could be, especially when it comes to making emotional decisions about things attached to people who mean a lot to me. But he was right. The next time, I started dedicating each weekly session to one or two rooms at a time and immediately started to see progress. Rooms were mostly empty after each visit. Now it felt manageable.

I removed the few things I wanted for myself. My favorite black dishes we only used on special occasions, the two brass giraffes that stood tall in the foyer, some of the artwork Mommy brought back from Africa, Egypt, and South America, the childhood portraits of me and my sister that had hung on the living room walls since 1971, and many other things that I held dear. Then I invited friends and family to walk through the house to take what they would cherish because they'd always remember it was once Mommy's. Things they had admired over the years, whether furniture, dishes, books, clothes, shoes, jewelry, electronics, or the pool table.

Clairees's sister, Doreen, was about Mommy's size. So, we went through all of Mommy's clothes, carefully selecting things that Doreen might like, but not too many because they had to be shipped to Atlanta. Some clothes still had tags on them, a reminder of the Mommy who bought things for their eventuality. She couldn't bear to be seen in the same outfit twice, and for that, she was amply prepared.

One Sunday, I met Ernestine and her other daughter, Kenni, at the house. Ernie was an important part of my support system, even though she saw her role as Mommy's protector. After the first stroke, Ernie chided me, telling me that it was my responsibility to do whatever my mother asked. Ernie had health problems of her own, and her daughters faithfully tended to her every need.

"I will never wash Mommy there," I remember vehemently blurting out one day when she and her family were visiting Mommy during her first acute rehab stay.

Ernie was right. I bathed and touched and cleaned up things that I never, ever thought I would, riding out yet another swell that could have overtaken me if I resisted.

The day Ernie and Kenni came, we spent more time talking and catching up than we did packing. We sat in the kitchen comparing caregiver experiences. Binky, Ernie's mother, a spry, vibrant woman who was a great-great-grandmother to many, needed someone to care for her. She could get around, but after her husband died, keeping her safe became a family priority. That responsibility fell mostly on Ernie, who conveniently for the others lived with Binky. Ernie felt trapped by her own health and the neglect by her sisters and brothers, who rarely relieved Ernie of caregiving, even though she needed it herself. They all seemed to go about their business, unwilling to share the load.

Kenni was Ernie's youngest daughter. She took after Ernie. Kenni was an extraordinary caregiver to her mother and her own children. No sacrifice was too big and no road to long to travel if family needed her. She and her sister, Nikki, were Ernie's rocks.

As we talked, I reminded Ernie that she has always been a nurturer. Caregiving was at the core of who she was. She babysat every child in her family and took in at least one that I knew of. She adored babies and children. Whenever she smelled a baby, it was like she had inhaled a drug. The genuine pleasure she got out of holding and cuddling babies was a powerful memory I held of her since I was a child watching her with her nieces and nephews.

I loved Ernie so much, and I wanted her to see herself as valuable, not as someone who had been left behind. In this special moment, I wanted to help her stop beating herself up for not becoming the things she dreamed of. I wanted her to see that she was living out her special purpose. She was, in many ways, not there by choice but by calling. She could be proud of that.

"Everyone doesn't think like you, Ernie. Your brothers and sisters aren't driven by the same forces that drive you," I said, trying to encourage her to let go of her anger and frustration. "It would be great if they did, but they don't. They won't, and there's nothing you can do about it."

I don't believe her siblings were being intentionally neglectful or mean. Their lives had taken them in different directions.

My words for Ernie were also meant for Kenni. Her tough exterior, I learned that day, was only out measured by her intense love for her family, especially for her mother. She and her sister, Nikki, who cleaned for my mother, saw Mommy as another mother, and for that I was lucky and grateful. I learned so much from the unwavering care they provided to the people they loved. They never questioned their place, but like many caregivers, they felt unappreciated.

Caregivers get so little credit for the Herculean tasks they take on every day. Instead, we celebrate stockbrokers, politicians, doctors, and lawyers. People who make a lot of money for the hardships they face. Family caregivers don't get paid with money, but I can only hope that their hearts are filled by knowing what they're doing is right, regardless of how little the world seems to notice. For me, Kenni's toughness was now forever softened by the knowledge that she was one of the kindest, most caring people I had the pleasure of knowing.

There are pros and cons to having someone else share the caregiving load. Although I had to care for Mommy all by myself, I found it liberating. I didn't have relatives with whom I could take issue if they didn't do as I thought they should. There were no family conferences. No conflicts around what was best for Mommy. No fights about money or what to do with the house. No scorn for how unevenly caregiving duties were performed. I was one hundred percent in control. I was the only person I had to convince at each fork in the road. I could ask for advice, but the final decision was mine.

I wondered often what it would have been like had Lynnette still been alive. There were times when I wished she was here to share the load. I imagined that we would have worked pretty harmoniously, caring for Mommy together even though she lived and worked in Pennsylvania.

We didn't get along at all as kids. We fought constantly just like typical siblings until she went away to college. As adults, that changed. We became friends. We were very different from one another, but we found common ground, things we enjoyed and could do together.

In my fantasy, I think we would have done well caring for Mommy. But then again, our relationship had never been tested like it would have been now. Would we have been able to devise a fair division of labor, one where neither of us felt put upon? Would we have been able to weather the emotional highs and lows of long-term caregiving? Would things long ago buried in our psyches resurface, causing the kind of rifts that takes other families to the brink?

Would that time I implied that she was lazy, embarrassing her in front my father's family, come back to haunt me? Or would I react to her many accusations that I was cold and unfeeling? That I was guilty of putting work before family? Would the fact that I lived closer to Mommy automatically mean I was to shoulder more responsibility? Would she use it as an excuse not to spend equal time meeting Mommy's needs?

There was also the fact that Mommy seemed to coddle Lynnette, giving her a free pass if she didn't want to spend her Saturdays working our family's flea market stand or helping Mommy with a project around the house when I was still single.

"She needs to spend time with her husband," Mommy would say. "You don't have anyone at home, so you need to be here." From my vantage point, Lynnette was Mommy's favorite. She treated

Lynnette with sympathy and understanding, while I always felt like I was held to a less compassionate standard than my sister, who dropped out of college, loved to party, and chose a simpler, noncorporate life. All that and so much more would probably have affected our caregiving relationship, but I'll never know.

Trying to control the way someone else fulfills their obligations gets mixed in with layers and years of family dynamics that can take the most levelheaded person to the breaking point. I was spared little else, but I was spared that.

CHAPTER 28

After one of Ernie and Kenni's trips to the house, I asked them if they wanted to visit Mommy. "I'd love to see Angel," Ernie said with characteristic dearness in her voice. We locked up the house, and they followed me in their car for the ten-minute trip to see her longtime buddy. Ernie's trouble walking meant the trip from the car, to the elevator, and all the way down the hall to Mommy's room was extremely taxing. Once we made it up to the third floor, she sat in the living room area closest to the elevator while I fetched Mommy.

"I have a surprise for you."

"Eminy?"

"Yep. And you're gonna love it. I brought someone to see you who will blow your mind."

I wheeled Mommy through the quiet halls to where Ernie and Kenni were waiting.

Her piercing laugh sliced through the silence like a hatchet through a wedding cake. She used her good foot to propel the wheelchair faster toward Ernie. They hugged. Mommy clasped Ernie's face, laughing and swaying back and forth. I had warned Ernie that Mommy's reaction was going to be way more animated than anything she'd ever experienced before. The woman who never let you know how happy she was to see you, who used sarcasm to water down her emotions, would be over the top.

This is how Mommy greeted everyone now. She couldn't hide her glee. It was as if all the emotion she had held back her entire life was now free to be fully expressed to everyone she loved. There was no containing it anymore. No more cucumber cool. No more side glances and measured welcomes. It was an all-out explosion of joy and excitement that sent shock waves through the air and down the hall.

She asked Ernie questions while I interpreted.

"Eminy?"

"How's Binky?" I asked as Mommy shook her head in agreement.

"Binky is fine," Ernie said with her signature deep-throated chuckle. "She's doing better than me."

"Eminy and Eminy?"

"How are Nikki and her kids?"

We went down the list. I knew Mommy so well that I could tell what she wanted to know from her friend that she hadn't spoken to since her second stroke.

She looked at me and said, "Eminy."

"You're welcome. I knew you'd want to see Ernie." She shook her head yes over and over. I had done good, and stroke had given me the late-in-life gift of my mother letting me know that what I did made her happy.

I called in an auction house, which was the next step in emptying Mommy's house. After I sent them pictures of what they could expect if they took the two-hour drive from Lancaster, Pennsylvania, they showed up with a truck and loaded it until there was no more space. They took anything they thought they could sell in an auction. The kitchen table and chairs, my sister's white lacquer twin bedroom set with two-sided panels in the headboards that could be switched from yellow to purple for a little color change, my lime-green and canary-yellow platform twin beds with open shelves and drawers, the matching yellow-and-green butterfly stand and glass top table. They took my parents' king-size bedroom set. The fake wood headboard was so dated that I just couldn't imagine anyone wanting it. I was happy that the experts saw it differently. It was now considered midcentury retro.

The men scoured the house, making sure they left nothing behind that could catch the eye of a bidder. It was hard to watch my early life being dismantled, packed up, and driven away by strangers. I took a photo and then watched the truck pull out of the driveway. Another of many sad goodbyes.

I filled dozens of trash bags, mostly with clothes that I decided had no more purpose, and left them on the front porch for Purple Heart. I'd go online at the end of each day of packing and request a pickup. It was tremendously convenient, which is what I absolutely needed at a time like this.

I chose Mondays to clean out the house because Tuesday was trash day. Clairees and I took the items left behind by friends, family, and auctioneers to the curb. The timing meant it wouldn't be out there for several days, signaling to the world that no one was home. Monday is also the day people in pickup trucks patrol neighborhoods looking for items to resell or turn in for cash. Whenever we'd take old broken, mildewed furniture, long-forgotten beat boxes, or old lamps to the curb, they'd disappear in mere minutes. It became a little game for Clair and I as we tried to guess what they would take or leave behind.

Some days, I'd catch them in the act, which would make their haul even sweeter. I'd invite them in and let them look around and take whatever met their criteria. Metals that could be melted down seemed to be a favorite, and Mommy had plenty of that in the way of old tools and store display parts.

One man even offered to buy my sister's 1997 Mitsubishi, which hadn't been road worthy for years and was now little more than a home to wayward bees. He came by one afternoon with a toolbox, cleaned it up, and got it started. He paid $250 in cash, which I put right into Mommy's bank account. Everything that sold, including what was sold at auction, meant another day, week, or month that Mommy could stay in lush comfort.

"Are you selling the Mercedes?" everyone from the auction staff, to men in trucks looking for metal, to the friends and family who came to help asked.

"Nope. My cousin is buying that. Sorry."

Clairees wanted that car, and I wanted her to have it. Mommy and Clairees adored each other. Clairees took on the one project I couldn't handle alone, and I wanted to reward her with the crowned jewel of Mommy's collection. I turned down offer after offer while she saved up the cash to buy it outright. She even paid to have it inspected and for the minor repairs that became necessary because that car sat unused for months at a time.

Friends with trucks pulled into the driveway every week, pledging to give new life to items that had long ago lost their luster. Most of the dining room set my parents bought when we lived in Philadelphia was split between Marci and her daughter, Val. I could look forward to seeing it each time I had dinner with them. I could be reminded of Mommy and many delightful family memories. Marci took the breakfront, which to this day conjures up images of where it stood in the dining room, what it was filled with, and how that room felt when it was crowded for Christmas or Thanksgiving dinner. Or the smoke-filled nights when Daddy played pinochle with family and friends. Or Daddy's excitement on that Christmas Day when he walked in the dining room to find the computer he desperately wanted sitting on the table.

Just like my grandmother, Mommy was tucking away cash in places I never thought to look. I got a call one evening from my neighbors Tim and Matt, who had gone to the house to pick up some things.

Tim called to tell me he found money in the cabinet behind the toilet in the master bathroom.

"How much?" I asked.

"I don't know, but it's all in hundred-dollar bills. Do you want me to bring it to you?"

"Absolutely!"

Shortly after, Tim dropped off seven one-hundred-dollar bills. All of which went right into the Paula wallet. That was the wallet I carried around with her cash to get her the things she requested or needed.

She had pretty much stopped eating the food being served. So every day, I'd stop somewhere I knew she loved to bring her something to eat. The money for every mocha milkshake, order of fast-food onion rings or turkey Reuben, her favorite pizza or crab cakes were paid for out of the Paula wallet. I even used it for the iPad she insisted that I buy her. She wanted a brand-new one. She insisted that a refurbished one wasn't good enough. But I went against her wishes, knowing she'd never be able to tell the difference.

After each house clearing day, I'd visit Mommy, never telling her what I was up to. I kept it a secret even though I didn't know if she'd be upset. The house had to go. There was nothing that could be done about it, and she didn't need to know that all that was once dear to her was waiting on the curb to be picked up by municipal trash trucks or being carted off by friends, family, and strangers.

I took a small risk that she'd figure it out by showing up one day with boxes and bags of photos. We'd sit in the living room area outside her room as she leafed through old photos and holding some up. With different inflections of "Eminy," she asked who was in the photo or where was the photo taken. We both enjoyed these brief trips down memory lane. The professionally shot pictures of Joanna and her sister, Regina, dressed in their fur collared coats, Sunday church hats, and heels. Photos of Uncle Jimmy and his military buddies or with a bunch of friends dressed to the nines on the Boardwalk in Atlantic City. It didn't matter how many times we had seen these photos before. It still felt so good to stumble across them again, like running into an old friend.

We'd laugh when I held up old pictures of our dog Pierre or react warmly when we came across photos of my cousins when they were small or pictures of family cookouts in our backyard. Throwing these memories away was inconceivable to both of us. They were all she and I had left of people, many of whom we had loved and lost. It represented another time that was filled with possibility, fellowship, love, and joy. Photos were often what made us stop what we were doing and smile, bringing us closer together when she and I were sharing the sad task of cleaning out the homes of loved ones passed. But sometimes, what we found revealed long-hidden deep pain and anguish.

When Mommy and I cleaned out Joanna's house, I found a letter from a woman with whom her second husband, Pete, had been having an affair. She called my grandmother horrible names, declaring that Pete didn't love Joanna and that she was a horrible person. These are the kinds of secrets children find out about when they're left to close out their parents' lives. Secrets they believed were buried deep enough that we'd never find them. Secrets that revealed the pain a loved one was experiencing behind the smiles they put on at the dinner table. Secrets you'd prefer to go to your own grave never knowing. Sadness, no matter how long ago, that still touches you deeply and forces you to make sense of how hard their life really was.

In that moment, I sensed how in their silence they showed their love. It was either love that made them hide these stories from us or sheer embarrassment of having botched things up so badly. Probably a little of both. But why did she hold on to such ugliness?

I felt sorry for Joanna. To learn that she had been the target of such vitriolic hate was hard to imagine. Even though she could be a difficult person, she was still my grandmother, and I found myself hoping that horrible things came to the woman who wrote these things. No matter how bad Joanna might have been, this woman had to be even worse.

I carefully placed the photos in brand-new photo albums that I found piled up in Mommy's upstairs hall closet and wondered if tying this project up in a pretty little package somehow signaled the end of her relationship with them. Once the photos were neatly tucked away on a shelf, our random encounters with them and the memories of these particular moments with these particular people were in danger of ending. In that way, her procrastination made sense. She wasn't ready to let go.

Six months after my cleanup project began, I met Alice at Mommy's house and signed the paperwork to put the house on the market. I stood in the empty house with my eyes closed and remembering the sound of Daddy's feet shuffling through the upstairs hallway in his favorite slippers with the broken-down backs to get a midnight snack. I could hear the console stereo in the family room playing Sunday morning gospel music on WDAS. I could hear Archie Bunker or George Jefferson's voices coming from the TV in Mommy and Daddy's room. I could hear Pierre barking as our visitors tried to leave. I could hear the muffled voices of Lynnette and her friends in her third-floor bedroom as they played Marvin Gaye and probably blew cigarette and pot smoke out of the window.

It was now nothing more than a shell filled with fading memories. Never again to host another Ruffin holiday or surprise birthday party. No more card games or surprise visits from the other side of the Ben Franklin Bridge. No more boyfriends stopping by or cousins spending the night, at least not for my family. After forty-three years, it was time to pass the baton to another family so they could start making memories here.

Against Alice's better judgment, we listed the house for $180,000. I knew I could always lower the price if it didn't sell, but if it sold instantly, I'd regret not having listed it for more. Prospective buyers responded swiftly to the low price in a very desirable community with a good school district. But the house was in such bad shape that many walked in and walked right back out.

About a week in, Alice called to tell me that a flipper was interested in the house. He was willing to pay $170,000 cash, which meant no mortgage financing to navigate and a quick settlement. I accepted the offer.

It was official. I had just sold my family home. Well, almost.

The lien search dropped more unfinished family business in my lap. Mommy and Daddy had taken a $40,000 loan out in 1987. It had been paid back. I knew that because in the two-and-a-half years that I'd been handling Mommy's personal business, no one came looking for the money. It turns out that amidst the shell game of bank sales and mortgage reassignments, the final paperwork never made it to the county office that tracks such transactions. The original bank that issued the loan was no longer in business, and the trail I was following had gone cold.

I'm convinced that this is the very reason so much family business goes unsettled. Why people walk away from valuable property. Why the streets of so many urban areas are littered with forgotten, boarded up, decaying homes. The system we must navigate is complicated, and today's gatekeepers aren't very helpful or knowledgeable. Business transactions are complex and unwieldy, making the option of walking away appear to be the best one.

I spent hours on the phone and online trying to piece together the facts and track down the status of the loan. I again sifted through the mountains of paperwork that were now at my house to search for loan documents. I had probably touched them at some point, but I didn't know they would be relevant. This is how one catches that "I'll just hang on to everything in case I need it someday" disease.

The house couldn't sell until this mess was cleared up, and the house had to sell to repay Abner's estate or else all of Mommy's savings, the money that was paying for her care and luxurious lodging, would have to be used to settle the family score.

I've always enjoyed untangling things. Give me a twisted wad of string and I will give you back a perfectly rolled sphere. Give me a puzzle and I will block everything out until I complete it. This was just another twisted wad that fate had handed me. But this was the kind of wad that involved other people, making it so much more challenging.

I was bounced around from bank to bank, department to department. I was told that this issue was not their responsibility. What they didn't understand was that I couldn't afford their no. What faced me if I failed was more than the paycheck they were struggling to earn. I told myself I was sticking this out for Mommy, not for me. Or was it for me? The consequences of Mommy losing everything was more than I was willing to accept. If I failed, she'd have to come live with me or go somewhere poorly managed or maintained. I was not walking away, even though I knew I would be walking away from a mistake that again wasn't mine or even my parents. I'd be walking away from the vision I had for my future.

I have fought enough battles to know that someone somewhere could fix this. Someone always can. My tenacity led me to a woman who could walk through the banking maze and navigate the regulatory requirements to which financial institutions must adhere. I had finally found someone with enough institutional knowledge to know what paths to go down. After a couple of trips to the county office to update the official records, the sale was back on track.

On September 18, the day that we should have been celebrating Lynnette's fifty-fifth birthday, I went to settlement and turned over a check for $154,000, closing out Mommy's debt.

It was a sad day, but I didn't cry. Two huge weights had been lifted. No more house and no more family crisis. I drove her precious Mercedes to my house and parked it at the curb, waiting for Clairees to buy it. She wanted to pay cash and was struggling to get enough together to pay what I knew the car was worth. Selling it for any less would mean less for Mommy's care. It was a beauty, and everyone who saw it asked to buy it, knowing it still had a lot of years left on it.

Fred grew impatient and goaded me into acting before Clairees's money came through. Eventually, we sold it to our tailor, who had admired it time and time again when he stopped by to pick up and drop off Fred's suits and shirts. He bought it and gave it to his wife as a gift.

CHAPTER 29

On the day I settled on Mommy's house, afterward, I picked up a milkshake and onion rings and went to see her. The living room area outside her room where she was sitting was dappled with early afternoon sunlight.

"Do you know what today is, Mommy?"

"No," she answered with one of the few real words she could speak.

"It's September 18, Lynnette's birthday."

Her eyes widened with surprise that she hadn't remembered that on her own.

I poured some of the milkshake into a Styrofoam cup, rationing it for the time when I wouldn't be there. She sipped the thick liquid out of the straw and put it down on the table while I removed puzzle pieces that one of her floor mates, who also enjoyed puzzles, had jammed into the wrong slots. I watched her do it with such glee, believing she had placed just the right piece. I didn't want to take away her joy. I waited until Mommy and I were the only ones at the table before removing them.

Each time I got a piece right, Mommy would smile, shake her head, and say, "Hun huh, hun huh, hun huh," congratulating me for the tiniest success.

"Mommy."

"Eminy?"

"I sold the house today."

She looked at me as if searching for something to say. And then she looked back to the television. That was it. No meltdown. No tears. She didn't even seem surprised. But I was. I had been withholding this for months, trying to spare her unnecessary heartbreak, but she was fine.

It had been a different scene the day I came by to pick her up for a cookout Ralph had invited us to. It was a graduation celebration for the daughter of an artist with whom Ralph had become close.

It was a great opportunity to get her out and into normal life in spite of my always present worry about navigating Mommy's wheelchair through a strange house. Ralph assured me that someone would greet us and help get Mommy inside. I also didn't know how they'd react to Mommy. We would be in a room filled with strangers that the old Mommy would have genuinely tried to get to know. All she'd be able to say now was "Eminy" and "No, no, no, no, no, no, no."

When I arrived to pick her up, Mommy was in her room watching TV and talking, as best she could, to her latest roommate. She looked at me and then behind me as if someone else was joining us. The week before, I had placed a picture on her nightstand of me, her, and Lynnette that was taken at one of my parents' friends' homes years ago.

Mommy rolled over to the photo and pointed to Lynnette and then looked back out into the hallway.

"Are you looking for Lynnette?" I asked with a thinly veiled look of concern.

"Hun huh."

"Do you have a sister?" her roommate asked.

"I did, but she died in 2002," I cautiously answered, splitting my glances between Mommy and her roommate.

In a flash, a wave of sadness took over Mommy's face. She looked at me as if she was hearing this for the first time. What was happening? Why, all of a sudden, does she not remember? Lynnette had been gone for over ten years, well before Mommy's strokes.

"Mommy, don't you remember? Lynnette had cancer. She's gone."

"No." She shook her head and began to cry. "No. No."

I sat on the bed next to her wheelchair. "I came to take you out today. We're going to meet Ralph at a cookout in Willingboro. Let's get ready."

"No," she said, tearfully backing away from me. The tears became steadier and more forceful. Mommy was melting down. She was inconsolably rocking back and forth, her good arm cradling her bad, lifeless arm, crying in a way I had never seen before.

I was confused. My heart was pounding. My mind was racing as I tried to find the right thing to say or do next. We had entered the twilight zone, where what I thought was reality was based on some unknown force. Was *this* her reality? Has Mommy believed all along that Lynnette was alive and just not visiting? Or had another stroke-related abnormality erased one of her most painful memories?

"Mommy, you'll feel better if we go to the cookout. Ralph will be there."

"No. Eminy." I took that to mean I don't want to go.

I began going through her closet, looking for something for her to wear. Each item I pulled out, she threw on the bed. I sat down, trying to keep my own emotions in check, and I waited. Over the next thirty minutes, Mommy's emotions stabilized, so I asked her again about the cookout.

"Eminy," she answered in a way that felt like she was saying "Let's go."

"Great. Ralph will be happy. He really wants you to come."

We changed her shirt, took a trip to the bathroom, combed her wig, and set off.

We were greeted by several people determined to help maneuver Mommy into the house. The family had moved their cars out of the driveway so we could park close. Several men and boys stood by eagerly waiting to help her transfer from the car, but just like a good mother hen, I waved them off and got Mommy safely into her wheelchair. The entourage followed Ralph as he wheeled her to the back of the house, and as other guests tried unsuccessfully not to stare, Ralph's squad of helpers lifted her over the lip of the back door and into a tiny family room.

That was where we would stay for our brief visit by Ruffin family standards. I fixed Mommy a plate of traditional cookout and family-made exotic island foods. I held her plate while she ate with her good hand. The food was delicious, but I was afraid that if she tasted something she didn't like, she wouldn't be able to hide it. I couldn't trust that her filters, the ones that governed the inner dialogue that used to tell her to eat it anyway, smile, and say how much you like it, would kick in.

Thankfully, she ate without incident, smiled her lopsided smile, and listened while I talked to the people around us. I tried to do what she would have done if she was healthy. I was the surrogate for the person who would make the new people we were meeting feel comfortable and important.

Those who knew her before approached us and said a few words. She nodded gleefully, showing how happy she was to see them. She'd cock her head toward me, a signal that I should introduce myself. Although everyone was gracious, I could sense uncomfortableness around having her there. She was handicapped, and people don't know what to say or do around someone who is handicapped. They couldn't ask why she kept saying "Eminy." They couldn't ask why she constantly tried to loosen the hand she held in a tight little ball. They couldn't ask why the woman who used to be the stately queen of style and glam was wearing nylon sweatpants and dirty, worn-out walking shoes. They couldn't engage in the kind of small talk that typically takes place at a party. They could only smile and nod if one of us caught their eye.

Had she been healthy, she would have been one of the women sitting at the kitchen table, getting to know one another. Or by Ralph's side as he buzzed about catching up with his friends and their family as they celebrated the high school graduate's milestone. But for Mommy, there would be no catching up. No making new friends. No celebrating or showing off that she was Ralph's squeeze.

We stayed for a couple of hours, honoring the invitation, the celebration, and the kindness of everyone we met that day. In the back of my head, I knew Mommy would have to go to the bathroom soon and that there was likely no space to maneuver her and her wheelchair into any bathroom in the small bungalow.

"It's been a long day, and I should get Mommy back." I was careful not to say where, even though anyone there who knew her knew her circumstances. Ralph would have certainly shared. But saying it out loud felt like it might have embarrassed her.

This was a rare moment where we were among people I didn't know and whose expectations of us I couldn't guess. I felt the pity of strangers. Instead of feeling grateful for their generosity, all I felt was hurt and sadness for Mommy. Another door was closing, the one that opened onto the glorious life she had, bouncing from party to party, collecting new people, and experiencing new adventures was over.

I drove her back to the facility and positioned her in front of the television in the living room area before heading home. It was a tough day on so many levels. One I just couldn't bear to repeat.

I kissed her cheek, said "I love you," and left as she settled into her movie.

CHAPTER 30

I became very calculating about where I'd take her and what well-meaning but impractical invitations we accepted. We did have some successful outings. I took her out to lunch for her seventy-second birthday. Ralph and her friend Albertha met us at The Italian Bistro in Marlton.

We sat outside on the patio overlooking the shopping center parking lot. It was a pleasant sunny day, and Mommy was happy about being the center of attention, the reason we were all together.

Ralph bought her seventy-two yellow roses, one for each of her years. He had also enlarged and framed a beautiful photo taken during their trip to Egypt. Like a king and his harem, Ralph sat on a thronelike chair with Mommy on his lap, surrounded by their friends and traveling companions. The friends were each holding their hands in prayer, the way servants would as they were about to bow to their king. In his lap was the queen, draped in a blue and white robelike gown with golden thread accents and matching pants. Her smile was rich, and her spirit was high. I had never seen this photo. Or if I had, I didn't remember it. She remembered, and it thrilled her.

We spent the afternoon together, her trying to speak and me interpreting. Sometimes Ralph, Albertha, and I would get into a conversation that she couldn't participate in, so she'd just stare off into space, waiting for attention to turn back toward her. Afterward, we took her doggy bag back to her room. Her appetite, even for the things she loved, had waned.

I had to enlist the help of the aides to find enough vases for all the flowers, which we placed throughout her room and the living room area. We even gave some to the nurses to decorate their office

221

space. I told them it was a gift from Mommy for all they had done for her, and in some ways, it was.

On another day, I took her sneaker shopping. She had admired one of the nurses' boldly colored running shoes. Each time Mommy saw her, she would point to her feet and say, "Hun hunh. Hun hunh. Eminy. Hun Hunh."

She had finally grown tired of the ratty walking shoes she had worn every day since her first stroke. She seemed to be overcoming her fear of taking risks, even the tiniest risk of wearing different shoes.

"You want a pair of those?" I asked.

"Yes!" She shook her head vigorously.

I loaded her into the car on a Sunday afternoon, and we went looking for new sneakers. We started at DSW in the nearby shopping center. I rolled her down two sneaker aisles slowly so she could browse the selection. Eventually, we found a pair of sneakers that must have had more colors than a rainbow. Yellow, purple, red, blue, green. This explosion of color was exactly what she wanted.

It was the first time we bought shoes for her in over two and a half years. Mommy had always been a size nine, so we started there. They were too small, and as I struggled to get them onto her feet, she erupted into an eardrum-piercing laugh that rang throughout the cavernous space. We were in the very back of the store in the clearance section, yet every head turned, from those close to us to the people at the register at the front of the store some one hundred feet away. I had become immune to Mommy laughing at my struggles. Sometimes I'd make a joke about her laughing at me. This time, I was embarrassed. We were getting the "Those damn loud black people" stares. Mommy didn't seem to notice.

We left there and went to the Moorestown Mall, checking every single store that carried women's sneakers, but we couldn't find the ones she liked at DSW or a suitable substitute. From there, we headed to JDR. It's similar to DSW in layout and selection. Eureka! We found the sneakers in the men's department. A men's ten, which is a women's size twelve. Mommy's feet appeared to have grown dramatically and mysteriously.

The day was not only an adventure back in time, but it gave Mommy something new to show off. No one could resist commenting on her wildly colorful new footwear. Each time, she'd smile hard, showing off how much she appreciated their compliments.

We began a spate of shopping and other adventures. We ventured out after she refused to wear two new wigs I bought her. We spent an afternoon at Lord & Taylor, shopping for clothes she insisted on buying but never wore.

The social worker was right. For the most part, we were now enjoying each other's company. Now we were just together, and it felt good. We were spending more time recreating than on meeting her basic needs. More and more, I was that eager parent dreaming up fun activities to my keep kid from getting bored.

When it was nice out, we'd sit by the pond on the property or walk around to see all the beautiful flowers brightening up the grounds. Or we'd go visit Mary on the second floor. That was until we got the sad news. Mary had passed away. The staff was afraid to tell Mommy until I was with her. They were kind enough to give me an address to send a condolence card. I signed Mommy's name, dutifully doing what I know she would have done if she could.

Even though my visits had become more social and less obligatory, I wasn't completely off the hook. Mommy was refusing to let the aides clean her dentures. Nor would she let the visiting podiatrist cut her toenails. Some of my visits were spent thoroughly cleaning caked-on denture plaque or pulling out the footbath I brought from her house to give her a pedicure. I'd wash her feet and paint her toenails, even though her feet were never exposed. Each time someone would come in to check on her and her roommate, she'd show off, grinning and nodding as if to say "My daughter is spoiling me." Sometimes, we'd go into the bathroom, shut the door, pull off her wig and detangle her real hair, moisturize her scalp, and twist fresh braids. Beneath her wig, her hair had thinned dramatically and had turned to spotty puffs of gray that knotted easily.

I looked forward to the two or three hours I spent with her every other night. Even though I was still serving her, I liked that it buoyed her spirit and that, even without words, she showed me she appreciated me.

There was such comfort in being with her. She was a presence I'd never been without. She was my mother. She was familiar and, for the most part, predictable and safe and mine. We belonged to each other. We shared that undefinable bond that would always keep me coming back. I guess you call that love.

One of our most interesting times together was the day Marci brought her therapy dog for what started as a normal visit. We sat in the living room area chatting while Marley, her gorgeous English Cream golden retriever, wandered about, sometimes into the room of one of Mommy's floor mates.

Suddenly Mommy's eyes lit up. She had an idea. "Eminy," she said, pointing down the hall. She was motioning in the direction of the birdcage, which was on the second floor.

"You want to take Marley to meet Sweetie?"

I'm not sure on what to blame my lack of good judgment. Maybe I was too distracted by Marci's and my conversation to think through what Mommy was asking. Maybe it was my reflex response to a Mommy request. Sometimes I'd find myself slipping back into "Mommy knows best" mode or the other excuse for turning off my reasoning skills—the "Her life's bad enough, I don't want to keep saying no, so I'll say yes to this" mode.

So Marci, Mommy, Marley, and I took the elevator to the second floor to visit Sweetie. As we approached the cage, Sweetie began chirping wildly at the seventy-pound predator that was marching toward her. Marley was on a leash, so Marci and I both assumed that would be enough to control Marley. But Marley pulled Marci hard and didn't stop until she was standing with both paws up on the wire birdcage, her hot breath panting into Sweetie's safe space. Instantly, Marci and I knew this was a huge mistake. She tried to pull Marley back, but the dog was winning the tug of war. Marley's single-mindedness gave her the brute strength needed to overcome Marci's five-foot-two frame as a small group of elderly residents watched, barely reacting as if they were having trouble registering what was going on.

I let go of Mommy's wheelchair and ran to Marci's aid. We both had a hold of Marley's leash, pulling with all our might. We fell to the floor, still holding on tight. Mommy sat in her wheelchair laughing hysterically. Her piercing laugh cut through the silence of the room, paralyzing the residents, who looked like they'd been hit by stun guns. Finally, Marci and I were able to stand back up and coordinate our bodies enough to pull Marley away and get her back on the elevator. I went back and retrieved Mommy while Marci negotiated with her dog, who had not given up on an encounter with Sweetie.

We rode the elevator with Marci to the first floor, where they got out and headed for the car.

"I guess that's the last time Marley will visit." I let out an exhausted sigh. Marci agreed.

I took Mommy back up to her room, silently hoping that no one had reported us. Mommy was still enjoying a good laugh about it, but it was hard for me to join her. Maybe that was her evil bird-hating plan all along. Befriend Sweetie and then get revenge on all bird-kind by having Marley eat Sweetie. I know that's not true, or at least I don't think it is. But her laugh was as diabolical as a super villain. I'll never know for sure.

CHAPTER 31

With Mommy safely nestled in a placed we trusted, Fred and I began to travel more freely. We celebrated our anniversary in St. Maarten. I checked in with Mommy every morning by phone and then enjoyed the rest of our days and nights worry-free. I tried to show her how to use FaceTime on her iPad, but that would have been a stretch before the stroke.

I bought her an electrifyingly red pullover top with matching pants that had the requisite elastic waistband. It was out of the question that I return from a vacation without a souvenir for her. It was rare that either of us brought the other gifts from our travels that the other liked. She always brought me something she thought I would like because she liked it. I always bought her something that she already had too many of. This time was no different.

For Mommy, it wasn't about the gift itself. Before the stroke, these trinkets were more about the pleasure she got from knowing my sister and I were thinking of her while we were away. I had come to believe these souvenirs were more of her self-absorption, but now I saw them as a symbol of our unbreakable bond. I wanted to think of her when I was away, and I wanted her to know it.

At first, she seemed excited about the outfit. I insisted that she wear it when we dined together for Mother's Day, but that was the only time it came out of her tightly packed closet.

In July, Fred decided to return to Montreal, our home away from home. After the debacle with Mrs. M walking out on Mommy in the middle of our last trip, we had decided to skip a year. This was our opportunity to get our tradition back on track. We stumbled onto the Montreal Jazz Festival in 1998 and looked forward to our biannual trips immensely. It was our home away from home and a much-needed respite.

When I informed the staff that we were going away, they asked us to consider having her complete a Physician Orders For Life-Sustaining Treatment or POLST form. It's not an advance directive, but in my absence, it would give those caring for Mommy some guidance on what to do if she had a health emergency.

We sat at the table as I read the document to her, asking the questions that I would mark with her answers. By this time, Mommy had stopped taking all her medications. Her feeding tube had been removed, and she was now free to decide what she would and wouldn't take. The nurses would come in and hold out their hands, which were filled with her meds. She'd point to each one.

"Eminy?"

"That's your blood thinner, which will lower your chance of having another stroke."

"No, no, no, no, no, no, no," she'd say, shaking her head to the rhythm of her words. Then she'd point to another one. "Eminy?"

"That pill keeps you from having seizures."

"No," she'd say and point to another one. "Eminy?"

"That one is for your diabetes."

Before answering, she'd cock her head to the side and give the nurse the kind of look that screamed "Are you kidding me?" Then she'd say no and turn back toward the TV, signaling that she was done with them and they could leave.

Dejected, the nurse and I would catch each other's eyes in silent acknowledgment. She had done what she was supposed to, and I was there to witness. There was nothing I could do to change Mommy's mind. She had graduated from taking the pills, waiting for the nurse to leave the room, and signaling me to hand her a tissue. She'd open her mouth and fish out the pills with her tongue to spit them out.

I'd then hunt down the nurse to get her more pills. We'd stand over her as she took them and then make her open her mouth and lift her tongue to make sure she had swallowed them. As humiliating as it might have been, she did it.

But she was clever and got much bolder once she figured out that I wasn't going to look the other way. Now, she just flat refused to take any medication.

Each time the nurses and medical staff would talk with me about this, they'd say, "Maybe she's given up. Maybe she's ready to go."

I couldn't hold back my chuckle as they looked at me with surprise. "Mommy isn't ready to die. She just thinks she knows better than you about what's good for her body." The day we filled out the POLST proved I was right.

"Mommy, I'm going to read the questions to you, okay?"

She shook her head yes.

"It says, 'Medical interventions: Person is breathing and/or has a pulse.'" Then I read the options to her. "Do you want full treatment? Do you want limited treatment or symptom treatment only?"

She rolled her eyes and glared hard at me. "Full treatment?" I asked.

She shook her head with a very definite yes.

"Got it. Next question. Artificially administered fluids and nutrition. No artificial nutrition, defined trial period of artificial nutrition, or long-term artificial nutrition?"

Again, her expression said "You know the answer, Kyle."

"Long-term artificial nutrition?"

Pursing her lips, she responded with a single nod.

"Okay. CPR. Attempt resuscitation? Do not attempt resuscitation?" I looked up from the paper to find her staring angrily back at me. "Attempt resuscitation it is."

"Eminy," she said in a way that could have been mistaken for nothing other than "Of course."

"Last question. Airway management. Intubate or use artificial ventilation? Do not intubate or something else?" I didn't look up. I just finished by saying, "I'm just asking the questions that are here on the page. Intubate, right?"

I could feel her glaring at the top of my head, waiting for me to look up to see the fury on her face. When I did, she looked into my eyes with such heated anger that I knew, without a doubt, that Mommy was not ready to die.

We continued our little outings. We couldn't go far, but we lived in a part of South Jersey that was constantly evolving. New buildings, stores, and houses were always in one stage or another of being built. There was plenty to show her within a few-mile drive. As we passed something new or a store that had changed hands, she'd stare out the window and point.

"Eminy?"

"Are you asking if that is new?"

"Eminy," she'd answer, shaking her head yes.

"Yes. That used to be a restaurant, but now it's an urgent care."

"Eminy," she'd respond, acknowledging that she understood.

One of her favorite stores on the planet was Loehmann's. I can remember as a child going to the store's cavernous fitting room with no booths or curtains. The Back Room housed designer clothes, some of which I'd categorize as haute couture. They didn't sell children's clothes back then, so for my sister and me, we had to entertain ourselves while Mommy scoured the entire store for unique finds.

Loehmann's had become a special place to Mommy, Fred, and me. We were all members in their frequent shopper's club, which meant added discounts around our birthdays. Every year before Mommy's stroke, we'd pick her up for a special shopping trip. It had become a tradition and a rare bonding opportunity for the three of us. Sometimes Mommy would buy our birthday presents if we were lucky enough to find something we liked.

Taking Mommy to Loehmann's now was an even bigger treat. I wheeled her through the racks, stopping whenever she reached out for something that caught her eye. At one point, she looked at me with panic on her face. She had to go to the bathroom, and we were in uncharted territory. When you're healthy and ambulatory, going to the bathroom in a place you frequent is a simple pit stop. You never stop to think about wheelchair access, transfer bars, or whether two people can fit in the handicap stall. Or even how much time you have before it's too late.

I recognized the look and began pushing her wheelchair toward the bathroom, but before we reached the door, Mommy grabbed my arm. When I stopped, I saw relief making its way across her brow. She couldn't hold it, but she seemed at peace with it. Her faith in the adult undergarment she was wearing was solid and true. She pointed behind me, signaling that she wanted to continue shopping rather than go to the bathroom.

"Okay, as long as you're okay."

She nodded yes.

We picked up a few cute things that I knew she'd never wear. She'd forget they were hanging in her closet, always choosing her go-to sweatpants and a small array of tops. Many times, she'd wear the same thing for several days. I think she was trying to spare me from doing her laundry so often, but I didn't mind. I had been doing her laundry since her very first acute rehab stay. I was in a groove.

On the drive back to the facility, Mommy got my attention, smiled her lopsided smile, and looked right into my eyes. With her good hand, she gave me a thumbs up. Shaking her head up and down, she said "Hunh huh, hunh huh." She couldn't have communicated her feelings more clearly with actual words.

On Wednesday of that very same week, an event I was planning for the Community Foundation of South Jersey was taking place at the facility that had become her temporary home. We were honoring a fellow board member in partnership with Symphony in C, a teaching orchestra that prepares professional artists for the orchestra stage. I arrived early to set things up and then went to Mommy's floor. I asked the aide to bring Mommy down to the ballroom so she could see the performance and see me in action. I wanted her to see for herself one of the projects I had been working on while taking care of her.

Amidst a room filled with distinguished businesspeople in suits, Mommy came in wearing her usual nylon sweats and a tight-fitting top that had shrunk and faded from being washed so many times. I was proud to have Mommy there. I introduced her to whomever I could in between making sure we stuck to our schedule. Since this was one of Fred's clients, he was there too. But there was one big hitch in the program that night.

The person we were honoring had just undergone emergency surgery at a hospital in Connecticut. My visit the day before turned into Mommy watching me put out this fire. She watched closely as I gathered input and led board members to our final conclusion. The show would go on.

It turned out to be a lovely evening for many reasons, most of all because I got to share it with Mommy. We sat together and watched the string quartet play oh so elegantly. Every now and then, I'd steal a glance at her. Her eyes were fixed on the stage, but she was showing little emotion. Classical music wasn't something that ever rose to the level of discussion in our family. I couldn't tell if she was enjoying it, and I wanted her to enjoy it.

When the performance ended, Mommy enthusiastically slapped her leg with her left hand. With her right arm paralyzed, it was the only way she could make a clapping sound. She had finally witnessed the fruits of my labor and met the kinds of people who respected and admired her daughter. I was her only remaining legacy, and I wanted her to revel in it. But more importantly, I wanted the people with whom I spent so much time planning this fundraiser to see where I came from. Even though on that night, Mommy was far from the glistening debutante I knew, I wanted them to meet the woman who was a big part of the person they believed they knew so well. Were it not for Mommy and Daddy, the indelible lessons they taught me, and the love and support they gave me, I would not have been confident enough to stand among them.

The following Friday, I visited Mommy as usual, but I broke the news to her that I would no longer be coming on weekends. I would be back on Monday. I was readying myself for the marathon ahead and decided it was time for Fred and me to enjoy full weekends, just the two of us.

"You're settled in and in good hands, Mommy. I think it's time."

She shot me a look of disappointment. Maybe it would have been better if I had not said anything. If I just didn't show up on

Sunday, would it have been less of a letdown than me announcing that I was abandoning her on weekends?

Visits from her friends had slowed even more. She built relationships as best she could with roommates who changed every few weeks. The staff knew her and treated her well, but there's nothing like a daughter's visit, and mine were surprisingly more cordial than some of the well-heeled daughters that came to see her roommates. Maybe it was because I had achieved a degree of peace with our situation. Or maybe it was because I didn't have children competing with my caregiving obligation. My flexible schedule allowed me to set aside time to spend with Mommy rather than running in, dropping off laundry, and resenting having to be there in the first place.

That day, Mommy resorted to the same thing she did every time I announced I was leaving. She'd look for little things for me to do that would keep me there. Get her ice cream from the kitchen. Put in a movie. Adjust the blanket that she carried like a two-year-old who found security in a random piece of fabric. Find the nurse to let her know that Mommy needed to go to the bathroom. Finally, she'd zone out, appearing to accept the fact that I was leaving, a passive-aggressive move that made it hard for me to say goodbye.

On this day, after I'd done as much as I was willing to, I slowly backed away from her and down the hallway while assuring her that everything she had asked for was in the works and that I would be back Monday.

I jetted out to my car and into a full, uninterrupted weekend of doing whatever Fred and I wanted. We probably didn't do anything that Saturday except go shopping, go to the supermarket, and watch TV while I drank wine and he enjoyed his favorite bourbon and a cigar. We settled in that night knowing that we could sleep in and still enjoy another full day of doing us. I felt a twinge of guilt, but not enough to choose Mommy over my marriage.

A ringing phone in the middle of the night does a better job of fully waking you up than a double-shot espresso. That night, my cellphone woke us up at about 2:00 a.m. Even though Mommy was in a safe place, I still kept it on my nightstand just in case. I answered before it fully registered that the news was inevitably bad. There are no good phone calls at 2:00 a.m.

It was the nurse on duty. "During my rounds, I found your mother lying in bed unresponsive. I couldn't wake her up. We already called to have her transported to the hospital."

"I'm on my way," I said calmly, partly from shock and partly because of the hour.

Once again, just as we had settled in to a nice, comfortable rhythm, here we were. I dressed quickly, grabbing the first thing I could put my hands on. Fred sprung out of bed and got ready to go with me. We pulled into the emergency room parking lot within minutes. Mommy's ambulance was arriving at the very same time.

Emergency rooms in the middle of the night are eerily quiet. The intensity of the daytime is noticeably absent. People who've been there during the day have either been admitted or sent home. It felt like we had the whole skeleton staff to ourselves.

The paramedics wheeled Mommy's gurney into a room as I stood by watching. She looked as if she was sleeping. I checked her chest for the rise and fall of her breath and was relieved when I saw proof that she was still with us. They didn't bother me for her insurance information. They just quietly hooked her up to machines and monitors and asked me to wait for the doctor.

Fred and I found places to sit in the tiny room while they shined lights in Mommy's eyes and cleaned away vomit, which indicated that she might have aspirated.

"Are you her daughter?" the nurse asked.

"Yes. Do you know what happened?"

"We don't know just yet. We won't know until we run a few tests."

They wheeled her out for a CAT scan, which, from experience, I knew wouldn't show a stroke for several hours, maybe even a couple of days. For the next few hours, all I could do was sit and look at her, hoping she'd open her eyes.

CHAPTER 32

The sun came up while we were in the ER. There were no windows, but activity around us began to increase, signaling a change of shifts and early morning arrivals. The results of the CAT scan were inconclusive. No one could tell us why Mommy laid before us unresponsive but breathing, and no one among the doctors, nurses, or technicians would chance a guess.

When Lynnette was diagnosed with lung cancer, people would ask about her prognosis, but we didn't have one. There was a time when it was common to hear something like "She has six months to live," but not in Lynnette's case. I never asked why they wouldn't give us a window. I assumed it was because of lawsuits that resulted from well-meaning people guessing incorrectly. But maybe it's because no one, not even a doctor, can really know exactly how long someone's body will withstand the ravages of disease. Everyone is different. God is the only being who can stamp an end date on someone. Or depending on what one believes, it's up to the myriad unseen forces that we as mere human beings may never fully understand.

They admitted Mommy midmorning, and we were ushered up to a room in the cardiac ICU. Fred and I sat comfortably in the large single room with her for much of the rest of the day. Updates were few and far between. It was Sunday, and in spite of health never punching a clock, hospitals function on a business schedule, ratcheting down on nights and weekends. It was quiet, and it seemed that mostly visitors passed by Mommy's door.

We were supposed to be leaving that Thursday for California with Marci and her family to run in a five-kilometer race through the Sonoma County vineyards. Instead, Fred went home and began cancelling yet another set of travel plans.

I couldn't hold it all in my head—what to do about Mommy while wondering whether things would be resolved before we were scheduled to leave. Cancelling it all was just easier. With that decision, I felt my load lighten.

I stayed until visiting hours ended. I had my computer with me and thought I might get some work done, but my heart wasn't in it. I returned on Monday and spent another full day sitting by Mommy's side. I had become pretty efficient about packing for a full day at the hospital. My computer, phone, iPad, and chargers were all I needed to feel connected to the world while locked away behind the glass cage of Mommy's ICU room. I spent very little time actually working, but having that option was my security blanket.

The doctors still had very little to report, but they continued to run tests to see if they could find the reason for Mommy's apparent coma.

On Tuesday morning, Fred and I arrived at the hospital around 10:00 a.m. I dropped my things off in the room and left briefly so I could talk to Clairees on the phone without disturbing Mommy. When I returned, a doctor was questioning Fred about his relationship to Mommy. The last thing that occurs to anyone who meets the three of us for the first time is that he might be her son-in-law. We're always put in the position of explaining that next to me, he is her next closest kin and someone with whom information can be shared.

The doctor asked us to follow him into another room, where he began to explain what they now knew. "Your mother has had another very serious stroke. We can't tell if the damage we're seeing is in addition to what was already there or evidence that the latest stroke has taken over an even larger area of her brain."

That news was sad, but not surprising. Mommy had been here before, and they had counted her out before. After the second stroke, they began to prepare me for the worst, and that was over a year ago. It was what he said next that made my knees buckle.

"She's not likely to come out of this coma. Essentially, she is brain dead."

Even if I suspected that, I wasn't ready to hear it. I wasn't ready to face the end, and I certainly wasn't ready to make decisions that were being asked of me.

The doctor continued, "Your mother is on life support, and that's the only thing keeping her alive. If we remove the breathing tube, we don't think she'll last very long. The decision about what to do is up to you."

I cried, and with each realization that popped into my head, I cried more.

My mother is about to die. She isn't ready to die. The day when we filled out the POLST, she asked that everything imaginable be done to save her life. Now I have to make the decision about waiting or nudging her toward the light.

"What would you do if this was one of your parents?" I asked the doctor.

I don't even remember what he said at that point. I couldn't take any more in. I had to make the hardest decision of my life. I was now in the very same situation that Mommy was in when her own mother was on life support. But Joanna was ninety years old. In the middle of the night, she called out to Mommy and then slipped into a strange state. It was like she was in a coma, but her eyes were open. She just kept gasping and gasping, her body jerking repeatedly. At the hospital, Mommy refused to let them remove life support. She insisted that Joanna would be fine, particularly since she'd been through so much and recovered before. Mommy didn't want to end it for Joanna, even though Joanna said she was ready to go right after her ninetieth birthday. She was proud of having reached that milestone, believing she had lived longer than anyone else in her family.

That very morning, Fred and I stood in the hallway with Joanna's doctor getting the details Mommy wasn't ready to hear. I asked the doctor if we could stop before she required heroic measures to keep her alive. I'd heard those words, even used those words, but I really didn't know what they meant, until the doctor answered.

"We're already taking heroic actions to keep her alive," he replied.

It then fell on me to convince my mother to let her mother die. "Mommy, the doctor said this is as good as Joanna will ever be. She can't recover from this, and the only thing keeping her alive is the machines." I tried to use reason to convince Mommy to let Joanna go. "Mommy, she's ready. The only person who isn't ready is you."

I never understood why Mommy refused to remove Joanna from the machines. They had a terrible relationship, always fighting. Neither wanted to be around the other, but Mommy's obsession with obligation was bigger than the two of them. Family is supposed to take on whatever they're dealt, no complaints, no shortcuts.

It was difficult for Mommy, but she finally agreed to remove Joanna from the ventilator. Joanna lived for another two hours before taking her final breath with her daughter dutifully by her side.

Now it was my turn. My mother and her fate were in my hands. It was up to me to wait it out for who knows how long before getting to the point where I truly believed she couldn't come back from this.

Countless people have to make this heartbreaking decision every day. This is one of those moments that TV and movies love to capture. There's a bit of romanticism around pulling the plug or making the decision to pull the plug. In the made-for-Lifetime movie playing out in my head, people are standing around Mommy's bed, sobbing uncontrollably. There's a minister pacing back and forth, bowing and praying for her peaceful entry to heaven. Loved ones are down on their knees, praying to God with the hand of a supportive friend or family member on their shoulder. Pulling the plug is drama at its best. After all, it is the moment we go from being into nothingness as far as we know. There should be drama, but in my case, there was just love, support, and a lot of waiting.

I decided to take the doctor's advice and remove Mommy from life support, but there were people I wanted by my side. I called Clairees, who came to the hospital with her brother, Jimmy. I called my cousin Denise, who also joined us, and Ralph, of course, I wanted there. I also called Mommy's loyal friends and travel companions, Violet and Albertha. No one wasted any time coming to our side.

The doctor said that once they removed the respirator, it might be a matter of minutes or even a few hours. Once everyone had arrived, I called the nurse into the room, and she gently pulled the respirator away, revealing Mommy's youthful skin and slender lips. We all held hands and circled around Mommy's bed, looking intently at her. Someone offered up a prayer. The heart monitor continued to beep as we all stared at Mommy, waiting for the moment of her peaceful departure. But Mommy wasn't ready.

For the next thirty minutes, our prayer circle remained intact. Then slowly, one by one, when it became clear that Mommy was stronger than the doctors predicted, the circle got smaller and smaller. As the sun began to set, the room started to clear, leaving only Clairees, Jimmy, and me. The three of us spent the entire night in Mommy's room, contorting ourselves into hospital room furniture, trying to get some rest, and listening as the beeps got further and further apart.

At one point, Mommy's breathing seemed labored, and then the death rattle set in. That gurgling sound that comes from deep in the chest signaling the heart is about to give up. The doctor had given the nurses permission to administer morphine to keep Mommy from suffering, and I took them up on their offer. Mommy's breaths slowed, and the heartbeats lessened over the next eighteen hours. Finally, the next morning at around 11:00 a.m., she took her last breath while I held her hand.

Shortly after she passed, Ralph and my cousin Judy arrived. We sat with Mommy as her body heat began to slowly dissipate. This was the first time I had ever been in the room with someone as they took their final breath. I wasn't there when my father, sister, or grandmother died. I couldn't even stand to be in the room when my first cat, Darby, was put to sleep. I didn't think I'd ever survive watching the life drain out of someone I loved.

I expected to feel much sadder, but I took comfort in knowing I had done everything I could for Mommy during the seemingly infinite struggles that followed her first stroke. I was truly at peace. I had looked after her and made sure she had the best care and attention. I sacrificed and stayed by her side up until the very end.

We had unexpectedly become closer than ever. I don't know if she had unfinished business with me, but I knew that I wanted no regrets when it was over. I still carried enough guilt and regret about not getting to tell Daddy how much I loved him. I carry regrets that my interference made Lynnette's final days more painful than they would have otherwise been.

With Mommy, I did and said everything I believed was in my power to do and say. I deceived her sometimes to save myself and to keep her from suffering more than she already had. I stepped back at times to let her take control of what was happening to her. In the end, I believe with all my heart that the decisions she made that led to her leaving this earth were hers.

I don't think she would have seen it that way. Her decision to stop taking her medications or give up on therapy was her way of controlling her life. Even when it felt wrong to me, I had to respect that she was my mother and she believed she understood the full picture. She was stubbornly trying to prove the doctors and me wrong. She had that right, but we weren't the villains. Her body was. Up until the first stroke, it had always been very good to her. Her only faults were her inability to accept that her body let her down and that modern medicine was the only solution.

I could have tried to force her to see it my way. But I would always be the naive daughter and she the all-knowing mother who was right even when she was wrong. That was a force I was powerless against.

CHAPTER 33

We laid Mommy to rest on October 31. Halloween is a holiday I never understood because it celebrates death and all things scary. I looked forward to the legitimate excuse to not open my door to strangers and their children.

Mommy was dressed in the ornate blue, white, and gold robe that she was wearing in the photo Ralph had given her on her last birthday. I was so glad we had bought her a new wig when we did. I couldn't bear knowing she'd spend eternity in a wig that looked more like a nest than hair. The day before the funeral, we inspected her body, and close friends and family came for a brief viewing. We were the only ones to see how beautiful she looked, but it didn't matter.

"You know your mother wants a closed casket, right?" Ernestine called to make sure I knew that Mommy had always insisted on a closed casket. Ernie needed to make sure I was planning to honor that wish.

I did know. "I don't want people staring down at me when I'm dead" is what she told me every time we left someone else's funeral. That was as close to planning for the end as we got.

I didn't follow the funeral template that Mommy carried in her head. I knew she had certain expectations about what funerals were supposed to be. Even though we never discussed hers, together we had planned or had been part of planning several. I asked her once what time someone's funeral was so I could plan to meet her there.

"Standard funeral time, Kyle," she answered with a high degree of disgust in her voice. I was supposed to know that viewings are from 9:00 to 11:00 a.m. followed by the 11:00 a.m. funeral.

Now the choice was mine, and I was making the final decisions for the person who taught me what it meant to be elegant, classy, and above all else, envied.

We held her funeral at the West Laurel Hill Cemetery chapel, which, unlike churches, limit how much time you can use their chapel. It was a small but elegant service and a far cry from the grand productions that marked Daddy's and Lynnette's farewells. Their funerals at Vine Memorial Baptist Church, our family's central place of worship going back generations, were attended by hundreds of people and lasted what felt like hours. But at West Laurel Hill, which is on the outskirts of the city as you enter the storied Main Line, there was a one-hour time limit. Still, the service was lovely and efficient.

Mommy loved going to church, but she didn't belong to one, so holding services and repast at Vine Memorial would have meant direct or indirect involvement by my Uncle Edgar, who I let word filter to that he was not invited to attend. Few from my father's side of the family came. The only Ruffins who were there were the ones who had been by my side throughout my caregiving journey. No other uncles, aunts, or cousins came. I just assumed that they were all out for my blood because of how Mommy had handled Uncle Abner's estate. Or that they were mad at me for banning Uncle Edgar and showing their solidarity by snubbing us.

But her loyal friends were there. So were old neighbors and longtime travel companions. And there was the lovely surprise of my friends who came because I lost someone dear. Not because of her but because of me.

So many shared their warm feelings about how well I took care of Mommy. I didn't expect to hear such compliments. Again, surprised by love, surprised that people were paying attention and that they felt compelled to let me know.

We buried Mommy in the plot I bought for my family in 1995 right after Daddy died. The day Daddy was buried, the family cemetery was showing its age, and I yearned for his final resting place to be as glorious as he was in my heart. I immediately bought the plot at West Laurel Hill and left it up to Mommy to have him moved so that ultimately we'd all be together. Instead, he remained buried in the old cemetery out by the Philadelphia airport and was now sharing the same plot as Joanna, his tormentor-in-law. I couldn't escape the notion that their spirits were in constant turmoil from living so close together for eternity. I pictured them bickering constantly as Joanna blamed him for everything bad that ever happened to my mother, including this. She would have found a reason to make Mommy's death Daddy's fault.

Daddy's parents and some if his siblings were there too. Mommy had decided that moving him would cost too much, so she didn't.

Most everyone who had attended the funeral drove the short distance up the hill to the family plot, past the mausoleums donning names of people after whom sections of Philadelphia and major city streets were named. It was a cool fall day, but the trees hadn't yet transitioned to their fall colors. The grounds were lush and perfectly manicured, and bouquets of flowers the cemetery placed on behalf of living loved ones dotted the landscape. The giant willow tree that once stood in front of our family plot—so large that you could see it from the road as you drove by—was gone and replaced with a new, gaited Jewish section of the cemetery. I chose this spot because of that tree. Its absence became another reminder that nothing is permanent. Just like each member of my family, the willow tree's time had expired.

As we sat by the graveside, Fred jokingly remarked, "You know, I only married you for your cemetery plot." We laughed a little, even though we were both sitting alongside the place where death would someday take us.

Lynnette was buried there, so at least mother and daughter would be together. Eventually, I completed my master plan and moved Daddy there too twenty years after he died. If Mommy was going to rest in this beautifully manicured place, so would my beloved father.

After Mommy's service, we held a repast in a nearby hotel ballroom instead of the usual church basement or community room. I had a chance to see people I hadn't seen for years and to thank those who had walked along side me at one point or another during my nearly three-year trek. It felt good to say "Thank you" but still strange to hear so many compliments about how well I served Mommy through it all. I think the stories Mommy had shared about me with her friends made them expect that I wouldn't rise to the occasion. That I'd find excuses to peddle her care off to others. Frankly, going in, I might have expected the same. But this test proved that I respected our mother and daughter bond. And yes, I loved my mother and miss her terribly.

If things were different, Daddy would have been leading the way all this time, trying to take on the full weight of Mommy's condition.

"Kyle, I need you to do me a favor," he might have called to say. "I have to go to work, and I need you to keep an eye on your mother until I get home." Only asking for help when he absolutely needed it. Or he might have repeatedly said, "Talk to your mother about taking her medicine and tell her to get off my back about taking mine."

I imagine Lynnette would have been by my side as I cleared out the house. We'd get into an argument because she'd arrive two hours late, a little buzzed, and with a girlfriend in tow. She'd work slowly and meticulously and become easily distracted over and over by old pictures or outfits that triggered memories. She would have left work and drove an hour to visit Mommy, bringing her food and sweets and keeping her up on the latest gossip. Her friends would have dropped by because they were truly special people and Mommy was important to them.

I tried to carry what I could of Daddy and Lynnette's loads. The person I was through it all—the person my whole family made me—couldn't have done things any other way. But I was about to learn a little more about who I was.

A few months after Mommy died, I got a text from a woman who said that my mother and her mother were sisters. I was completely perplexed. All I could think was that Joanna could not have had more children without me knowing. My mother so completely distanced us from our grandfather, her father, that his connection never occurred to me. Once it did and she began sending me photos of my grandfather, her grandmother, and her mother, I was astonished.

For the first time, I saw the person whose nose and complexion I inherited. Colonel was his name. He was tall and handsome and appeared to have led a full life after he divorced Joanna. She sent me a picture of her mother, and quickly I saw how much she resembled Lynnette.

I didn't know if my grandfather was still alive or how old he was when he died or if he was the reason Mommy had strokes. Was it in her genes? Was it in mine? A big part of my family puzzle was filling in, and for that, I was grateful.

What I lost when Mommy died was so complicated. She filled a space in my life that I took for granted. I saw the world through her. She shaped my perception of so many things.

When I got my first cat, Darby, I brought her to Mommy and Daddy's so she wouldn't be alone in my apartment while I was at work. Darby was a Calico, and I wasn't familiar with Calico markings. I thought she was hideous.

"Isn't she ugly, Mommy? She's all splotchy and random," I said. It didn't matter. She was a found kitten discovered in a public park in Philadelphia, and I was keeping her.

"She's not ugly, Kyle. She's adorable. Look at those big, bright eyes. She's cute," Mommy sweetly replied. In an instant, Darby changed to my eyes. It was as if Mommy had cast a spell on me. I now saw Darby the way Mommy saw her.

It happened again when Fred and I got our cats, Tortie and Kaylee. I could see their beauty, but it was Mommy who pointed out how soft they were. And suddenly I could feel Tortie's cottony softness and Kaylee in all her silkiness. Mommy could magically shift my awareness, allowing me to see and feel beauty that was hidden from me. She showed me how to appreciate things that were different, and I never gave her credit for that.

Some of life's best gifts you don't ask for. You can't pick them out of a catalog or from a website. They don't cost money. They come from unexpected places. When you get this kind of gift, it becomes a permanent part of you. It seems harsh to call Mommy's stroke a gift, but it brought us closer than we'd ever been. She finally got the doting daughter she wanted. I got a loving and appreciative mother, the one who was buried beneath the layers of the life she had been dealt. Even though her words had left her, she told me loud and clear.

Mommy's and my story isn't big, sexy, or filled with grand accomplishments, abuse, neglect, or even riches. There were no harrowing adventures or complicated mysteries. Our story is the same as so many people who commit to caring for another because they can't imagine doing anything else. They are unsung and not rewarded nearly enough for what they sacrifice. But their stories are real and repeated over and over.

This was the book I was searching for after Mommy's first stroke. The one in which I could see myself. The one that could shed even the tiniest light on how stroke would change my life. I couldn't find it, so I wrote it. What's your story?

ABOUT THE AUTHOR

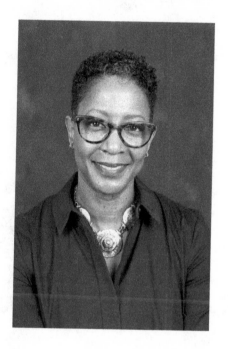

Kyle Ruffin is a marketing and communications consultant who has had a long career working in the media and nonprofit fields in the Greater Philadelphia region. *In Stroke's Shadow* is her first book, which she views as an important tool for opening up conversations around the impact of caregiving, particularly for African Americans.

Serving as the only family caregiver for her mother who suffered three strokes had a lasting impact on her. And when others began coming to her for advice after finding themselves in the same situation, caring for a loved one after a stroke, she knew sharing her story could help others feel less alone of their journeys.

Kyle is a dynamic speaker and presenter, who has now turned her attention to talking and writing about caregiving to help others see this role as a calling rather than a sentence. She knows how isolating caregiving can feel, and she seeks to help others connect, heal, and embrace self-care.

Learn more about her at mycaregiverstory.com or follow her on Facebook and Instagram at @mycaregiverstory.

Kyle lives in South Jersey.

CPSIA information can be obtained
at www.ICGtesting.com
Printed in the USA
BVHW082329110122
625986BV00001B/99